naming bebe

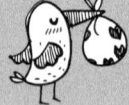

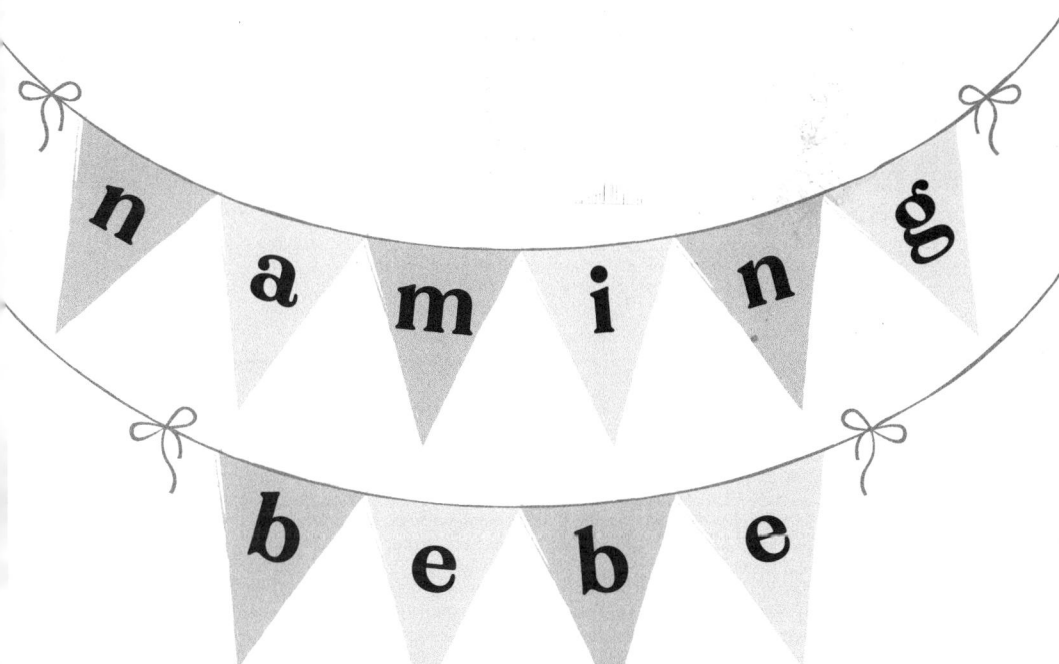

naming bebe

An Interactive Guide to
Choosing a Baby Name You Love

Colleen Slagen

Tarcher
an imprint of Penguin Random House
New York

Tarcher

an imprint of Penguin Random House LLC
1745 Broadway, New York, NY 10019
penguinrandomhouse.com

Most Tarcher books are available at a discount when purchased in quantity for sales promotions or corporate use. Special editions, which include personalized covers, excerpts, and corporate imprints, can be created when purchased in large quantities. For more information, please e-mail specialmarkets@penguinrandomhouse.com. Your local bookstore can also assist with discounted bulk purchases using the Penguin Random House corporate Business-to-Business program. For assistance in locating a participating retailer, e-mail B2B@penguinrandomhouse.com.

Book design by Laura K. Corless
Interior art: baby illustrations © notkoo / Shutterstock.com

Library of Congress Cataloging-in-Publication Data

Names: Slagen, Colleen, author.
Title: Naming bebe: an interactive guide to choosing a baby name you love / Colleen Slagen.
Description: New York: Tarcher, 2025.
Identifiers: LCCN 2024040352 (print) | LCCN 2024040353 (ebook) |
ISBN 9780593719121 (trade paperback) | ISBN 9780593719138 (epub)
Subjects: LCSH: Names, Personal.
Classification: LCC CS2367 .S53 2025 (print) | LCC CS2367 (ebook) |
DDC 929.4—dc23/eng/20241213
LC record available at https://lccn.loc.gov/2024040352
LC ebook record available at https://lccn.loc.gov/2024040353

Printed in the United States of America
1st Printing

The authorized representative in the EU for product safety and compliance is Penguin Random House Ireland, Morrison Chambers, 32 Nassau Street, Dublin D02 YH68, Ireland, https://eu-contact.penguin.ie.

For Rory, Janie, and George,
a joy to name and a joy to love.

And for Dan,
my biggest supporter through this whole adventure
and not a bad namer himself.

contents

introduction ix

PART ONE
how to name your baby . . 1

1. Goals 3
2. Style 17
3. Popularity 43
4. Family Ties 67
5. Common Quandaries 81
6. Choose a Name 105

PART TWO
name inspiration . . 115

acknowledgments 207
notes 209

introduction

So you have a baby on the way. Your mother-in-law thinks Ellen would be a nice name (her name is Ellen). You told Grandma you were thinking of using River, and she ended up hospitalized for a week. Your friends think Olivia is too popular and you should choose something more unique. The internet told you Noah is a boy name, don't use it. You were set on Josephine, but your sister-in-law beat you to it. You pivot to Lucy, but your husband knew a girl named Lucy in fourth grade and vaguely remembers her being kind of mean. He uses his fifty-third veto.

Let's turn off the noise. It's time to find the baby name that's perfect for you. Welcome to your modern-day baby name guide! By the time you finish this book, you'll have both an abundance of name inspiration and full confidence in your ability to pick the perfect name for your child.

I've been a name nerd for as long as I can remember. What did you like to do as a kid? Take your Razor scooter for a ride through the neighborhood, perfect your cat's cradle, tenderly care for your American Girl doll? While you were doing that, I was reading all the names listed in phone books. And yearbooks. And movie credits. And obituaries (is that not what they're for?). I used my diaries to invent families so I could name people; my first entry is from 1997, when I was eight years old. On a trip to a bookstore with my best friend's family in middle school, while my friend and her sisters picked up copies of *Gossip Girl*, I spent my money on *Beyond Jennifer and Jason*, a baby name book that became my name bible. And I forced *everyone* to talk baby names with me. Lucky for me, a lot of my family members were also baby-name-curious, and we spent vacations having roundtable discussions about baby names, which got even more exciting (and relevant) when there were actually pregnant family members.

When I grew up and my friends started having kids, I naturally started doing name consultations for the ones who were willing to humor me. I received some very positive feedback, and with a little encouragement from my optimistic and entrepreneurial husband, I created a website at the end of 2021. I pitched it to some local mom groups on Facebook and started getting some real clients. By this time, baby name consultants were starting to become "a thing" on social media. With two young kids, a job as a nurse practitioner, and some stage fright, I thought I'd keep it as more of a hobby. But in early 2023, I mustered the confidence to post a few videos on TikTok as @NamingBebe, sharing some consultations I had done. I started a series called "Names I Can't Use," where I picked names that commenters liked but couldn't use and suggested similar alternatives. Before I knew it, I was going viral.

I soon began spending every naptime, weekend, and sacred hour after the kids went to bed working on baby name consultations and content. I began getting featured on outlets like ABC News, Fox, *Today*, *Glamour* magazine, Business Insider, and NPR. By August 2023, I decided to go full-time as a baby name consultant. It was not an easy decision after all I'd invested in my career as a nurse practitioner, but I felt like I was one of the lucky few who had the opportunity to turn my passion into my job and I would have been crazy not to see it through. No, I didn't study baby names in school (though if that had been a college major, I would've had summa cum laude in the bag), but I have developed an expertise. I spend my days talking about baby names, reading forums, poring over data, and analyzing trends. I have an endless index of names living rent-free in my head (taking the place of other important details). As of this writing, I've helped hundreds of families choose a name for their child.

It is not lost on me that when families hire me as a consultant, they're trusting me to be a part of a very intimate and personal decision. It's not "just a name." It's really the first label you're bestowing upon your child, one of the first and most prominent pieces of their identity. For a lot of people, hiring a baby name consultant takes a leap of faith. It might seem like a strange concept, and they're not sure exactly what to expect. But my clients routinely tell me that they're blown away by the detail and consideration that goes into their consultations and that having a third party weigh in alleviated so much of the stress that can cloud the process. I feel incredibly grateful that I get to help families with this decision. And with this book, I'm putting my expertise directly in your hands.

Far too much parenting these days is done without a village. It's a lot of stress on parents! When you read this book, I hope you'll relate to the challenges and delights other parents are experiencing when choosing a baby name. This book will be your baby-naming village; a place for you to see yourself in the stories of other families.

This book is not just a big dictionary-style list of names (though it does include plenty of name inspiration—see Part Two: Name Inspiration on page 115). Rather, it's an interactive guide that will let you apply my tried-and-true methods to your own process. A variety of exercises and journal prompts will help you explore your name preferences, with real-life sample consultations woven throughout. As you work your way through the book, you may want to pause and take some time to do a little research at points.

Feel free to flip back and forth to the name inspiration in Part Two whenever you see fit. Do the activities you find helpful and skip the ones you don't. In the end, there's no right way to do it, and you'll figure out how this tool best serves you.

Yes, naming a baby can be stressful, but it's also special—and fun! Whether you're coming to this process with a blank slate or you've been keeping a running list of names on your phone for years, my hope is that this book will provide you with the information, tools, and space you need to help drown out the modern-day noise and restore joy, creativity, and simplicity to the naming process. Once your child is born, they'll imbue their name with meaning, and you'll never look back!

how to name your baby

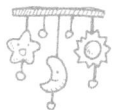

Welcome to your modern guide to naming your baby! Part One of this book will walk you through every part of the baby-naming process, from establishing your goals to looking at data-driven trends to finally settling on a name. Along the way, you'll consider style, sound, popularity, and more, aided by plenty of exercises to help you explore your options. We'll even dive into the solutions to some common issues, like choosing complementary names for siblings. And don't forget—you can flip to Part Two: Name Inspiration on page 115 at any point to see lists of potential names organized by your favorite aesthetics.

·1·

Goals

We've been engaging in the act of naming for millennia. Although practices and traditions have changed over the years (I'm not sure how many of Adam and Eve's friends were called Maverick), names have always been a significant part of our identity and culture.

A name is important, and the fact that you're reading this book shows you know that. Our names are often the first things someone learns about us: the first opportunity for connection—and the first opportunity for judgment. The name you choose for your child feels like it could be a prophetic declaration of who they'll become. Will they be an artist or a CEO? Quiet and demure, or animated and unfiltered? Could Birdie be taken seriously in a boardroom? Will Cornelius get bullied at school? Parents feel the burden of this decision and how it will impact their unborn child's future.

What makes a name "good"? This is subjective, and everyone is going to bring their own experiences and associations to the discussion. What you think makes a successful name someone else may find uninspiring. A name you find professional someone else may find snobby. There is no objectively perfect name—it's all about choosing the perfect name *for you*.

You're already doing the work of putting thought and care into your child's name, so when those anxieties start to creep in, remember that your child will also be so much more than their name. Of course, that's easier said than done, but that's where this book comes in.

Naming Bebe will thoroughly explore the ins and outs of naming a child—emotions, aesthetics, practical matters, and more. We'll look at every aspect of the naming process, from popularity to phonetics to family traditions. By the end, you'll go into the delivery room with full confidence that you can select the perfect name for your child! In this chapter, we'll start by setting goals and laying out the framework for your naming journey. (And if you want to browse name lists while you're reading, don't forget you can flip to Part Two: Name Inspiration at any time!)

Let's start with an exercise that will help you think about names in practical, personal terms by considering what your name has meant to you over the course of your life. Maybe you grew up as Nate and hate that you had to write Nathaniel on all your forms. Maybe you grew up as a Sara and they spelled it *S-a-r-a-h* on one too many Starbucks lattes. Maybe you were always known as Lauren C. and don't want the same fate for your daughter. Either way, you probably have some feelings about your own name.

What is your name? _____

Do you like your name?

Circle one: *Yes*   *No*   *It's fine*

If yes, what about it did you like growing up? What about it do you like as an adult?

_____

_____

_____

_____

_____

If no, what do you not like about it? Does this give you an idea of some characteristics you do/do not want in the name you choose for your child?

_____

_____

_____

_____

_____

Modern-Day Baby Naming

Wouldn't it be easier if we could just go back to 1950 and name all our girls Linda, Susan, or Nancy and all our boys Robert, Richard, or Gary? Maybe, but it would also be such a snooze! In 1950, roughly 50 percent of baby boys had one of the top 20 most common names—that's a *lot* of Michaels and Davids. Compare that to 2023, when only about 15 percent of baby boys have names in the top 20. Modern naming has given us the courage to embrace more unique names! We have a greater appreciation for individuality today, and this is very much reflected in the fact that people are giving their children names like Banks, Clementine, and Dove.

In fact, names like these have become so popular, you might even say having a unique name is no longer . . . unique. This is evident both anecdotally, as we come across more unique names in our daily encounters, and in the data, as we see the top names being used with less frequency than they were thirty years ago. This is often a reflection of parents' values and aspirations for their children. Rather than wanting their child to blend in and not get teased for being different, they hope to be a family who celebrates being creative and special. It's also a phenomenon that has sort of a domino effect. When people see that unique names are more culturally acceptable, it emboldens them to act on an impulse toward nonconformity—or simply to have more fun with baby naming and veer away from traditional norms and cultural, religious, or family expectations.

Before social media, I bet the naming process was much easier. When our parents and grandparents were naming kids, they had no idea that Susie from high school also named her daughter Emily, so they didn't feel they had to avoid that name. Their exposure to names was much more a product of their intimate circle of friends, family, and community, as opposed to the two thousand people we follow today on social media. I've had so many women message me to say things like "My mom named me Jessica/Amanda/Ashley because she loved the name and had never met one before." Now, we see a name used once by someone we don't even plan on talking to for the remainder of our lives, and somehow it loses its novelty or feels "used."

Along with all the names we're now exposed to, announcing your baby's name has become something like a personal style statement for everyone to judge. You've got the custom-engraved oak name sign to place next to your baby's tiny hand in their social media debut. The oversize banner conspicuously hung over the crib for the nursery-reveal photo. A whimsical yarn crown embroidered with your child's name for their first birthday party. It feels like the whole world is waiting on the other side of your phone, ready to critique your choice. And you can't return those Etsy purchases. This adds an element of perceived pressure and consumerization to the naming process that didn't exist at this scale before social media.

Names are also more visible than ever before, literally and figuratively. In prior generations, our experience of a name was more auditory—it was spoken aloud far more often than it was written. But with modern technology, our identities are embedded in the visual medium of writing, permanently and constantly displayed in social media profiles, dating profiles, email addresses, and so on. In the past, your résumé with your name at the top was viewed by only a handful of people throughout your life. Now, it's publicly available on LinkedIn for everyone to see. I heard a story years ago of a woman who claimed the Gmail handle for her child's name before she was even pregnant. This type of next-level planning might not be common, but it does speak to a whole different set of concerns facing modern parents during the naming process.

On top of that, census data tabulating all the names given to babies in the United States every year is now easily accessible online. So whether you're a name nerd who refreshes your browser obsessively around Mother's Day (when the previous year's name data typically gets published) or just a normal person who finds themselves reading a puff piece on the topic over your morning latte, there's a good chance you're familiar with the most popular names for girls and boys in any given year.

The majority of clients I work with want a compromise: a name that both stands out *and* fits in. They don't want their child to have three other kids in their class with the same name, but they also don't want their child to go through life saying their name and getting a confused look in response or having to clarify pronunciation and spelling in every interaction they have. So while I see people gravitating toward more unique options, practicality remains important too.

We think of names as being more conformist in the past, but there have been plenty of times in history where unique names were in vogue. Puritans in seventeenth-century America gave their children names like Remember, Experience, Fear-not, and Joy-in-Sorrow. By that metric, you could argue that modern "virtue names" like Sincere and Serenity are actually quite traditional!

What hopes and fears do you have about choosing a name for your baby? Are you feeling excited about getting creative? Stressed out by the pressure of finding the perfect name?

_____

_____

_____

_____

_____

_____

_____

_____

Intuitive vs. Practical Namers

I divide parents-to-be into two general camps: intuitive namers and practical namers. Intuitive namers tend to seek out a name that is more unique or whimsical, that holds special meaning or significance, or that somehow matches the energy of the child they're expecting, such as a song title or a place-name they've associated with the pregnancy. Practical namers, on the other hand, think more about logistics: pronunciation, spelling, name flow, popularity data, and trendiness. Both approaches—or a blend of the two—are totally valid.

Some people come to me with very specific goals: "We want a two-to-three-syllable feminine name that's outside the top 100 and has a built-in nickname option." Others aren't sure where to start and want help exploring all their options. Whether you want a name that has been around for thousands of years or something that feels fresh and modern, identifying what kind of namer you are may help you establish your naming goals and priorities! And whatever those goals and priorities are, this book will help you achieve them.

List five qualities that are important to you in a name. Are you more of a practical namer or an intuitive namer?

_____

_____

_____

_____

A Sample Consultation

In a moment, you'll get to start thinking about your naming goals in detail. But first, I want to show you a sample consultation (edited for clarity and length) so you can get a better feel for what my process as a professional consultant looks like from start to finish.

This is a consultation for one of the first clients I ever worked with. This couple had had an easy time naming their first child, Grace, but were struggling to find a name for their second child. They had a few names they liked, but nothing felt like a slam dunk in the same way Grace had. They had already put a lot of thought into the name and came to me with lots of different criteria and potential meaningful connections they wanted to incorporate.

Here's the wish list they gave me:

- Top contender: Philippa, with nickname Pippa. Dad loves more than Mom. Name of a favorite book character.
- Other contenders: Zoe, Willa, Louise, and Madeleine
- Middle names: Elizabeth, Dove, or Irene
- Mom likes/Dad vetoed: Sasha, Dora, Corinne
- Dad likes/Mom vetoed: Abigail, Charlotte, Sophia
- Can't use: Esme, Maeve, Juliet, Christine, Aisling, Roisin
- Names they like but that feel "too big": Wilhelmina, Willela, Winifred, Theodora

- No names that end in a long *ee* sound
- Bonus for a name that contains a bit of both parents' cultures (Irish and Jewish)
- Prefer traditionally feminine names as opposed to unisex
- Like names with a family connection and/or names from favorite book/TV series (Dune, The Locked Tomb, *The Expanse*).
- Mom likes names with a positive connotation from the Hebrew Bible or a botanical connection
- Dad likes names from Greek mythology
- Family names include Elizabeth, Doris, Estelle, and Irene, and the initials B, R, or L

I started by giving them commentary on their wish list and highlighting a few alternative names that were similar to ones on their list. For example, Iris has a similar feel to Willa, has a floral connection, and comes from Greek mythology (the goddess of the rainbow). The name Corinne felt too out-dated for one partner, but I suggested Cora as a similar and more modern-sounding alternative that also had a Greek mythology connection (another name for Persephone). I also provided an exhaustive list of different forms of the name Elizabeth that could be used to honor it as a family name while still being unique, as well as a list of names that mean "star" to honor the family name Estelle.

After many hours of research, here are some of the names I recommended for them:

- **Margot:** Not only a stylistic match but also a character in Dune. It's a familiar but uncommon name and has vintage, feminine appeal.

- **Seraphine/Seraphina:** This name comes from the Hebrew Bible but also fits your naming style with its feminine, whimsical, artistic aesthetic. Sadie would make a cute nickname (Sadie is a nickname for Sarah, thus the connection). Seraphine/a has the creativity of some of the names you felt you couldn't use, like Willela, but I think the biblical connection makes it feel more accessible and the nickname Sadie pairs well with Grace.

- **Quinn:** A short and sweet name that has Irish roots *and* is a character in the Locked Tomb series. While it is a more unisex name, it's ranked number 85 for girls and number 440 for boys, so much more often used with girls.

- **Eilis/Eilish:** This name is an Irish variant of Elizabeth (pronunciation can be AY-lish or EYE-lish). The phonetics are beautiful, and it's a way to tie in both the Irish and Hebrew connections, as well as family significance honoring Elizabeth.

- **Selene/Celine:** A timeless feminine name, with Cece, Lena, or Leni as nickname options. Selene is the Greek goddess of the moon, and this name gives a nod to Grandma Estelle with the shared celestial meaning in both names ("moon" and "star").

- **Daphne:** Daphne has a connection to Greek mythology as well as a botanical connection in its meaning: "laurel tree." Its timeless sophistication makes it a great match with Grace. It is familiar but not often heard (ranks at number 415). Daphne Dove would be a stunning combination honoring Doris, or consider Daphne Elise for something more traditional in the middle that honors Elizabeth.

- **Beatrice:** While this name doesn't have any significance to the many connections you named, it struck me as a name that may fit your style. It pairs well with your last name and has a sweet nickname in Bea. It's unique but traditional, quirky but polished, and is uncommon but becoming more mainstream (it has gone from number 970 in 2000 to number 550 in 2020).

- **Selah:** Selah (pronounced SAY-luh or SELL-uh) is a beautiful, simple, albeit unique, name with Hebrew origin (it's a word used in the Bible to indicate a pause or moment of reflection after a musical sequence).

This couple ended up picking the gorgeous name Daphne Elise, going with a name that felt familiar but uncommon and contained a connection that was meaningful to each of them!

Now it's your turn! Let's go over your most basic goals.

Are you looking for a first name only, or a middle name too?

First only   First and middle   Middle only

Are you naming one baby or more than one?

1   2   3+

Do you know the sex of the baby?

Girl   Boy   Don't know

Do you and/or your partner have any names in mind right now? (If you don't, don't worry, this book will help you come up with plenty of great options.) If you do, write them down here. Don't hold back—write ALL your options, even the ones that seem unlikely. Even if you don't end up choosing any of them, they may help you figure out what you want and don't want in a name. And remember that writing names down here doesn't set them in stone. You may be in a completely different place by the end of the book—or you may end up close to where you started but confident it's what you want.

Girl	Boy

No, really, write ALL your options! What are your Hail Marys? Names that maybe you haven't said out loud because you assume they're an automatic no. Maybe they give you imposter syndrome. Have your partner write their Hail Marys too.

Girl	Boy

What are some names that you and your partner agree on, even loosely? (If the answer is none, don't panic. That will change by the end of this book!)

Girl	Boy

What are some names you love but can't use for whatever reason (a cousin is already using it, it's the name of your ex-boyfriend, etc.)? These, coupled with the names on your list above, can help you home in on your style and explore other names within that same style.

Girl	Boy

Buckle In

Now that you have your creative naming juices flowing and a few basic goals in mind, it's time to start thinking about details! In the next chapter, I'll discuss popularity, aesthetics, meaning, name flow, and more—with lots and lots of examples to help you zero in on the perfect name and advice on navigating some of the most common dilemmas parents face when choosing a name. Remember: Your goals are your goals. Whether you want something traditional or modern, quirky or common, you will find the perfect name *for you*. And have fun!

· 2 ·

Style

One of the most important aspects of a name is simply its style. How does it look when you write it? How does it sound when you say it? How does it make you feel when you hear it? For most of us, hearing certain names can instantly conjure up a specific image or stereotype. Maybe Ashley is captain of the cheerleading squad, while August is soft and sensitive. Perhaps Franklin has his library card's ID number memorized and Hattie is home-schooled on a farm in rural Vermont. Cody Campbell will definitely be a famous quarterback when he grows up.

As a name consultant who thinks about names all day (and, more frequently than I'd like, in the middle of the night), I of course have my own preferences when it comes to phonetics, sibling name cohesion, and other elements of style, which I'll include. But I'm here to help you select a name that suits *your* preferences. This chapter will help you explore the sound, feel, and overall style of different names.

This is also a good time to remind one partner (there's always one) that it's important to keep an open mind. Instead of instantly throwing out a veto like it's a red card at the World Cup, let some names marinate for a while, and don't be afraid to explore options that may feel a little outside your comfort zone. There are a lot of things we don't love the first time we experience them—songs, fashion trends, even personalities—that grow on us over time.

Aesthetic

Do you prefer something traditional or something more modern? Something sweet or something sophisticated? Something casual or formal? I find it helpful to categorize names under different aesthetics. A "cottagecore" name, for example, evokes the simple romance of farm life—think Mabel or Polly for a girl, Edwin or Ernest for a boy. A "quiet luxury" name, on the other hand, is sophisticated and classy, perhaps reminiscent of British royalty, like Arthur or Stuart for a boy or Beatrice or Alice for a girl. Floral-inspired names, Bible-inspired names, Italian names—all of these aesthetic categories can be helpful to think about when choosing what your child will be called. Some aesthetics are more trendy, while some are more timeless.

Perhaps you like the established, classic feel of using a surname as a first name. I remember back in the 1990s when Rosie O'Donnell used the name Parker for her son and I thought, *What was she thinking?* Parker is now in the top 100 names for boys and number 115 for girls. Rosie, I never should've doubted you! I love when parents are open to surnames as first names, because it opens up so many possibilities. You can really take this style in so many different aesthetic directions! You could go with what I call an "old soul" surname like Abbott or Clarke or a more "old money"–sounding surname like Kennedy or Wellesley. You could pick something that matches your family's heritage (Murphy or Sullivan if you're Irish) or even incorporate an aspirational figure (Jagger or Hendrix if you like classic rock). It's all a matter of your personal taste.

Personal taste is, of course, subjective. You may think Wyatt is a rugged cowboy name while your partner thinks it's vintage and preppy. But having worked with hundreds of families (and having talked and read endlessly about names), I find that if you give me a name you like, I have a pretty good idea of what other names you might also like. My first viral video on TikTok was part of a series I still do called "Names I Can't Use," in which I ask viewers to comment with a name they love but can't use, and I'll give them the perfect alternative. For example, if you like but can't use the name Vivian, you might want to go with Scarlett, Eloise, Genevieve, Penelope, Charlotte, Margot, Georgia, Daphne, or Florence. If you can't use the name Sloane, you may like Reese, Blair, Blake, Shay, Maeve, Eden, Collins, Quinn, Rowan, Sawyer, or Arden. This concept of understanding your style and pinpointing similar alternatives is the foundation of my consultations.

Whether you want something short and crisp or long and frilly, your aesthetic preference is one of the most important factors in choosing a name. This is why Part Two: Name Inspiration is organized by aesthetic category instead of alphabetically: to help you zero in on your personal style and group your favorites together.

If you could give a label to the style of name you're looking for, what would it be? Think of this as a brainstorm and write down anything that comes to mind—they could be well-established styles you've heard of (vintage, nature-inspired), something more creative (gentle lumberjack or Bridgerton-inspired), or just general adjectives (cute, rugged, romantic). Then consult Part Two: Name Inspiration on page 115 and see if any of the categories there come close to the categories you've created. If so, they may be a good place to start!

_____

_____

_____

_____

_____

Gender

Traditionally, we divide names into "boy names" and "girl names," but as gender norms and roles are changing culturally, naming choices are following suit. This is not an entirely new phenomenon—many of us knew both boy and girl Sams or Alexes or Taylors growing up—but now we see a lot more fluidity, with more names being used equally for both genders and some names strongly associated with one gender being used for the opposite gender. Rihanna named her son Riot Rose, while Chrissy Teigen and John Legend gave their son the name Wren; both Rose and Wren are typically used for girls. On the other side of the equation, Blake Lively and Ryan Reynolds named a daughter James, while Kylie and Jason Kelce used Wyatt, Elliotte, and Bennett for their daughters. These are names that are common for one gender and don't even rank inside the top 1,000 for the opposite gender—at least, not yet.

While I think this is slowly starting to evolve, people are generally willing to push the boundaries further for girls in terms of breaking tradition and crossing typical gender lines. Parents have always seemed to be willing to get more creative and adventurous with girl names while preferring something more established and masculine for boys. I think this is because, consciously or not, we tend to see boy names as strong and powerful, qualities many have come to view as positive in little girls, whereas girl names are more likely to sound soft or sensitive, qualities that are sometimes stigmatized in males.

Surnames that have become popular as first names for boys, like Carter and Parker, are now being used for girls, as are what I call "my best friend's dad" nicknames like Scottie and Stevie, and even very traditional boy names like Spencer and Logan. Some parents are attracted to the effortlessly cool aesthetic they feel gender-neutral or traditionally male names give to their daughters. Some also see it as giving their daughter an advantage in a world that often favors men. The stereotypes that come to mind when meeting— or hiring—a girl named Rowan or Drew might be totally different from those associated with a sweeter or more proper-sounding name like Charlotte or Abigail.

Some parents sidestep the issue entirely by gravitating toward names with gender-neutral nicknames, which feel flexible and inclusive. I recently did a consultation for a couple who were attracted to frilly feminine names like Aurelia, but one of their stipulations was that the name must have a gender-neutral nickname option. I'm seeing this more and more—feminine names that have boyish nickname options (like Francesca to Frankie or Eleanor to Leni), or vice versa, masculine names with girlish nickname options (like Elliott to Ellie).

Again, this is more common when naming girls than when naming boys, but I think this speaks to an overarching theme of both cautious creativity and name versatility. Choosing a name like Francesca with Frankie as a nickname gives your child options. When they're old enough to have opinions on how they want to present themselves to the world, they can choose something more playful or something more formal, something feminine or something more masculine. Regardless of your reason, being open to gender-neutral names expands your name pool and allows for more creativity. Flip to page 139 for gender-neutral names, page 132 for feminine names with gender-neutral nicknames, and page 152 for masculine/gender-neutral names with feminine nicknames.

There is a long history of names starting out as male names but gradually becoming more common as female names over time. The names Allison, Leslie, Ashley, Lindsay, and Meredith were previously used almost exclusively for boys before becoming almost universally used for girls.

Do you want a name that's masculine, feminine, or neutral? Why?

_____

_____

_____

_____

_____

Meaning

Did you know that Cameron means "crooked nose," Amara means "eternal beauty," and Mallory means "unlucky"? Some names have obvious meanings in English, like Grace, Summer, or new-on-the-scene Ransom. Some names mean something in other languages that we might not speak, like Nathaniel (Hebrew for "gift from God") or Khalil (Arabic for "friend"). While I think that, for some people, the meaning of the names they like is secondary, if it's even a consideration at all, exploring names with specific meanings or connections to certain values or ideals can be a great way to find inspiration.

I worked with one couple who were in search of a boy's name that was strong and masculine, ideally with a meaning related to animals or mountains. Their top contenders were Magnus and Ari, and they liked but had ruled out Aldous, Aaron, Leo, Atlas, Max, and Rex. My list of recommendations included the following:

- **Rafe:** an Old Norse name meaning "counsel to the wolf"
- **Anders:** a Scandinavian name meaning "brave and manly"
- **Berg:** a German name meaning "mountain"
- **Merrick:** a Welsh name meaning "power" or "fame"
- **Barrett:** an English surname meaning "bear-like"
- **Evren:** a Turkish name meaning "dragon"
- **Adler:** an English name meaning "eagle"
- **Lennox:** a Scottish name meaning "with many elm trees" (mountain-adjacent)

They ended up choosing Anders; they loved the strong meaning and they were particularly drawn to A names. If you have a specific meaning or value—like hope or happiness or strength—that you'd like to incorporate in the name you choose, you can do research online or call in a name consultant to help you find a name that both suits your style and has a significant meaning. For a list of girl and boy names with positive meanings, flip to page 170.

Does the meaning of your child's name matter to you? Circle one.

It matters a lot   It might matter somewhat   It doesn't matter

If you have some top name contenders right now, do you know what they mean? Try Googling to find out and write the results here.

Name	Meaning

Do you have any strongly held values or ideals you might want to incorporate into your baby's name? If you don't plan to use a family name in the middle, this can be a great place for a name that feels slightly out of your comfort zone for a first name! Write some here.

_____

_____

_____

_____

_____

Now Google "names that mean [meaning]," filling in the values or ideals you wrote above. If any results appeal to you, write them here, alongside their meaning.

Name	Meaning

Ease of Pronunciation

For some parents, ease of pronunciation is nonnegotiable. They don't want their child to experience the inconvenience of having to correct people their whole lives or wonder if it will impact every first impression. Where this ranks in priority when choosing a name is often a product of our own experiences.

While choosing a more mainstream or traditional name (William, Katherine) is one way to guarantee easy pronunciation, there are also less common names that are phonetically intuitive, especially surnames like Banks or word names like Maple. Conversely, there are some fairly mainstream names for which you'll likely need to clarify pronunciation, either because there are multiple correct pronunciations (Vera can be VEER-uh or VARE-uh) or because they're not necessarily phonetically intuitive (Esme, Rhys). These are lovely names! Just because ease of pronunciation is important for some parents, it doesn't have to be a priority for you.

Phonetics

Phonetics are the sounds that a word makes when you say it out loud. Think back to ninth-grade English class. Remember assonance (repeating a vowel sound, as in "rude blue lagoon") or consonance (repeating a consonant sound, as in "cracking back")? How about alliteration (starting multiple words with the same sound, as in "softly, silently swooning") or rhyme (ending multiple words with the same sound, as in "loud crowd")?

I don't mean to make choosing your child's name as painful as a high school homework assignment, but phonetic elements like these can make a name sound melodic, poetic, or just plain memorable. Think of the alliteration of Case Keenum (a former NFL quarterback, of course), the assonance and near-rhyme of Conan O'Brien, or the consonance of Jackson Pollock.

Consider the names that stick with you. There may be sounds you're attracted to in a name without even realizing it!

Most often, the parents I work with assert preferences about whether a name is more cacophonous or euphonious—strong-sounding or soft-sounding. Beck or Knox, for example, have a much different phonetic feel than August or Silas, and these differences impact the vibe the name evokes. Knox might feel more masculine, crisp, and strong, while Silas might feel gentle, sensitive, and thoughtful. Picture the type of person who might use these sorts of names. A bookstore owner may gravitate toward Silas, while a navy pilot may go with Knox.

Are there any letters or sounds you want to avoid? (For example, maybe your older child's name starts with R and you don't want "matching" names.) List them here.

_____

_____

_____

Are there any letters or sounds you particularly favor? (For example, maybe you love names that start with J or end with an ee sound.) List them here.

_____

_____

_____

Length

How long should your child's name be? I find people's preference is often a product of (a) their experience with their own name, and (b) cohesion between a first name and a last name. Someone with a name like Alexandria probably either grew up casting a scornful glare toward anyone who tried to shorten her distinguished, five-syllable name to Alex, or she absolutely hated the inconvenience and will now name her daughter Elle. For the most part, parents with a longer last name prefer to balance it out with a one- or two-syllable first name, and parents with a one-syllable last name prefer at least two syllables in the first name for optimal flow. There is nothing inherently wrong with a name like Cam Rhodes, but it sounds more staccato than, say, Carson Rhodes, which has a more natural meter that alternates between stressed and unstressed syllables.

Overall, shorter names tend to feel lighter and more effortless, which gives them a cool or chic vibe. They can also feel more straightforward and less susceptible to being altered or nicknamed. Longer names can have a more elegant or decorated feel and often (but not always) lend themselves to nicknames.

Think about if you named your child Charlie as opposed to Charles. Charlie feels friendly and casual, while Charles feels distinguished and regal. But of course, these are not absolute rules. For example, Leo is quite short and Oliver is longer, yet these two names share a similar vibe.

How long do you want your child's first name to be? Circle one.

1 syllable   *2 syllables*   *3 syllables*

4+ syllables   *People really care about this stuff?*

Spelling

When you give your child a name, you're not just choosing how that name will be pronounced, you're also choosing how it will be spelled—and some parents get very creative with spelling. If you look at the top 1,000 names, you'll see several names that are alternative spellings of one another. For example, *five* different spellings of the name Charlie rank in the top 1,000 for girls: Charlie, Charley, Charli, Charlee, and Charleigh. For some names, there has long been more than one accepted spelling, like with Rachel and Rachael or Katherine and Catherine. But with the rise of invented names and a trend toward wanting a more unique moniker for your child, it has become more common to change the ending of a name from an -ly to a -lee or -leigh (Kayley/Kaylee/Kayleigh) or to change a more traditional ending of -ton to a -tyn (Peyton/Peytyn).

If you ask me, a unique spelling does not a unique name make. Spelling the name Elena as Alaynah, with a *Y* and an *H*, may look more distinctive, but when the teacher reads through the class list, no one will know the difference. Intentionally going with a nontraditional spelling solely for the purpose of trying to make the name more special sets your child up for a lifetime of correcting baristas and fruitlessly searching for their name on a key chain at the souvenir shop.

That said, many people would disagree with me here, as evidenced by the data. One argument in favor of spelling a name differently is that, more and more, the spelling of our names is highly visible via email addresses, social media handles, and so on. In a sea of Elenas on the company-wide Zoom meeting, the Alaynah in your little square may set you apart.

Will This Name Embarrass My Child?

No one wants to give their child a name other kids will tease them for. As someone who was called Colleenie Weenie (primarily by my siblings), I would be remiss to ignore this topic. Are kids on the playground today still saying Smelly Ellie or Hairy Mary? I'd like to think we are raising a more open-minded generation of children, and given that the current generation is gravitating toward more unique names, nontraditional names certainly stand out less than they used to. Kids are used to hearing a range of names and are less fazed by hearing a name they haven't heard before. I barely turn my head now when I hear someone shout the name Archimedes or Lavender at the playground.

One thing I would still consider is your child's initials. There are a lot of three-letter words or abbreviations that would be less than ideal to have as your initials. I once had a client whose first-choice name had the initials IBS, and she had to think hard about how important it was to use a family name that started with B as a middle name. (This one I advised against.) There is no need to overthink this, though. I remember talking to a friend who was worried that her son's initials were going to be the acronym for a rare genetic disorder. I assured her very few people would even register that.

Some name teasing will likely always be a part of childhood, but I think there is far less risk that your child will get made fun of simply for the fact that their name is unique. You can't predict what other children (or, unfortunately, immature adults) will find funny or weird. Should you be prepared to get some comments from the grandmother behind you in the grocery store line if she hears you calling your child Aspen? Probably. Overall, however—and I hope this isn't an overly optimistic take—this is not a concern that I would put too much stock in.

Nicknames

Nicknames are one of the most common ways we express affection and familiarity. Some names have well-established nicknames, like Ted for Theodore or Maddie for Madeline. Other names don't have well-established nicknames or end up lending themselves to a more unpredictable nickname (e.g., shortening Christopher to Chip instead of Chris, or shortening Alexander to Xander instead of Alex). Some established nicknames don't make much intuitive sense, like Peggy for Margaret or Hank for Henry. In any case, potential nicknames are an important consideration during the naming process.

For the most part, there are two groups of namers: those who love nicknames and want to plan accordingly, and those who don't understand why you wouldn't name your child what you plan to call them. (The latter are often the Allies and Bens of the world who wish their birth certificate didn't say Allison or Benjamin.) Personally, I'm a nickname lover. I tend to gravitate toward names that are playful and friendly, but I'm a traditionalist at heart and prefer a more formal given name. My daughter, Jane, goes by the nickname Janie in everyday life; my son Rory has earned a slew of nicknames in our household through a series of ridiculous rhymes and associations with his actual name. We plan for our youngest, George, to go by George, but we love to endearingly call him Georgie too.

In an era of creative naming, I find a lot of people are interested in a more formal given name with great nickname potential, like Calvin to Cal or Vinny, or Penelope to Penny, Poppy, Nellie, Lo, or even Pepper. As a name consultant, I love that nicknames are a way to get creative when working with strict naming criteria, like trying to incorporate a family name. They can also be a great way to compromise between two partners who have different naming preferences, as well as a way to get cautiously creative with a name while retaining a formal/traditional name to fall back on.

You may be asking, "Can't I just name my son Charlie instead of Charles?" Of course! This is a completely personal preference and a growing trend—names like Millie and Ellie actually rank in the top 150 for girls now. Some parents have concerns that these names aren't professional enough, but I think that notion is outdated. By the time your child enters the workforce, they'll likely be submitting their résumé to someone who's a millennial or younger and is used to hearing all kinds of unique names. In a world where people can wear athleisure to the office, I don't think having a résumé that says Ellie instead of Eleanor is going to keep anyone from getting a job.

On the flipside, a common concern is parents who are attracted to a name but not its nicknames. Can Madeline avoid getting called Maddie? Can William avoid becoming Will or Billy? I think this is somewhat name-dependent. For some reason, Carolines are able to remain Caroline, not become Carrie, but Madelines will almost inevitably be Maddie to someone. It's also child-dependent. While you can correct people and ensure your son is called Robert and not Rob, at some point, you can't really control what your child prefers or what friends call them, so parents should be prepared to relinquish some control.

I recently worked with a client who wanted to use the name Kit for her daughter but was very concerned that she would spend her entire life carrying around an air horn to blow anytime anyone dared to call her Kitty. To her, Kitty felt like an overbearing, high-society mother-in-law, while Kit was cool, crisp, and modern. This is a case where I think most people would not use Kitty unless they heard the parents use it, but of course, adding -y or -ie to the end of a name is one of the most common ways to create a nickname. If you are firmly anti-nickname, I would try to find a name that doesn't have a super common natural nickname, like Noah as opposed to Samuel, or Violet as opposed to Penelope.

Another common request I get is from parents who love a certain nickname but don't love the most obvious associated formal name(s)—they like Emmy as a nickname but not Emma/Emilia/Emily as a given name. You could certainly use Emmy on its own, but there are also a lot of less conventional options for a given name that allow for Emmy as a nickname, such as Emmeline, Emerson, Emery, Emmett, Gemma, Esme, Ember, Emerald, and Clementine. You could even choose a first and middle name with the initials

M. E., like Maeve Elizabeth or Matilda Eden, to get the nickname Emmy. It depends how creative you're willing to get, but if there's a nickname you love, it's worth doing research to find a formal name option you love just as much!

I worked with one couple who knew they were going to give their child the nickname Rocky, a family name. For a son, they planned to use the obvious given name of Rocco, but they found themselves quite stuck when they learned the baby was a girl. They considered Rochelle, Rockwell, and Brooke but didn't love any of them. I separated their recommendations into three different categories: names that could sensibly nickname to Rocky (Roxanne, Veronica, Rachel); names that arrived at the nickname Rocky by pairing an *r* sound in the first name with a *k* sound in the middle name (Rooney Kaia, Ruby Lachlan, Rose Pollock); and names with a meaning tied to rocks, stones, or gems (Alaina, Halston, Gemma, Jade). (I loved the idea of getting the nickname Rocky from the literal meaning of her name!)

In the end, they planned to go with Ruby Lachlan . . . but after seeing her in the delivery room, they felt the name Rocky didn't fit her at all, did a complete 180, and went with Maxie Rose. It's rare, but sometimes couples make spontaneous name decisions that are right for them!

Do you want to give your child a name that will be nicknamed?

Yes   *No*   *I could go either way*

If you have certain names in mind, write them here and list potential nicknames.

Name: _____

Potential nicknames: _____

_____

Name: _____

Potential nicknames: _____

_____

Name: _____

Potential nicknames: _____

_____

Of the nicknames you listed, are there any you particularly like or dislike that would rule a given name in or out?

_____

_____

_____

_____

_____

On the flipside, if you have a nickname you plan to use, like Rocky, what are some creative formal names that could plausibly use that nickname? (If you don't want to do your own research, this would be a great question for a name consultant!)

_____

_____

_____

_____

_____

_____

Middle Names

Middle names are kind of like those ice makers that make ice in the shape of nuggets instead of cubes: They're not strictly necessary, but they can be fun or elevate a beverage—or, in this case, a name. Think about your current peers and friends you've made as an adult. Do you know their middle names? (I admit I do, but I'm not a good example. "What's your middle name?" comes before "How are you?" in my conversations!)

Even if they don't usually have much day-to-day importance, however, middle names are a fantastic place to honor a family member or to have a little fun, picking a name that's out of your first-name comfort zone. Some people are looking for a middle name that provides balance and versatility. If they want to give their daughter a gender-neutral or masculine-leaning first name like Sawyer, they may look for something more traditional and feminine in the middle like Mae. If they're choosing a unique family name for their son like Winston, they may choose something more mainstream in the middle like Lucas. This way, in the rare situation that the first name doesn't suit the child (or they become a famous musician), there is already an alternative in place.

In a generation of parents who grew up with 80 percent of their friend group having the middle name Marie or Elizabeth or Nicole, some middle-name diversity is appealing. In fact, I have a lot more interest in middle-name consultations than I ever expected! Now that social media has us displaying a baby's first and middle name on clothing, birth announcement signs, nursery banners, and more, middle names are getting more attention. Fewer people are feeling the pressure to continue family traditions (like giving every daughter the middle name Anne) in favor of choosing a middle name that they love just as much as their first-name choice.

I worked with clients who were interested in "stunning" first/middle name combinations that felt whimsical and nature-inspired. They wanted a variety of pairings, some more feminine, some gender-neutral. Some names on their list included Bloom, Wren, Magnolia, Dovie, Arlie, and Navy. Here are the name recommendations I gave them:

- Ivy Rain
- River Isolde
- Marigold Lucy
- Briar Bea
- Jovie Wilder
- Coco June
- Scottie Sage
- Elodie Fern
- Luna Love

- Pepper June
- Isla Seraphine
- Kaia Marlowe
- Stella Blue
- Story Jane
- Tallulah Capri
- Winslet Prue
- Soleil Clementine
- Daisy Frances

They chose the beautiful combination of Soleil Winslet. They were drawn to both the meaning (Soleil means "sun" and Winslet means "joyful dwelling") as well as the matching s and l sounds in both names. A romantic, whimsical, and meaningful combination for their first child!

Of course, what's considered cohesive is subjective. Some people love the sound of a name like Elena Isabella—feminine and elegant with ending syllables that echo each other—while others may find it a matchy mouthful. One-syllable middle names have a sleek sound and phenomenal flow with most first names. From classics like Claire or John to sweet vintage names like June or George to more modern options like Sage or Rhodes, they work well for both girls and boys. (This is part of why a major trend right now is using James as a middle name for girls: Amelia James, Vivian James, Merritt James, Ivy James.)

I myself have gravitated toward using family names in the middle and have prioritized that over a first and middle name that flow perfectly. I recently had clients who wanted to use the name Kimberly in the middle, after an aunt who had passed away, even though it didn't align closely with their taste and didn't have the best flow with some of their top first-name contenders. While you could get creative (use Kay instead of Kimberly, for example), that just didn't feel as significant as using the name the aunt was known by. I fully support prioritizing an honor name in the middle over perfect flow, and that's what they ended up doing!

The most important takeaway with choosing a middle name is not to let that decision steal the show. While it's nice to picture a beautiful three-name combination on your child's future save-the-date, don't make a choice based on the occasional scenario. In day-to-day life, it's their first name they're going to be using.

I only have one big middle-name caveat: Don't use your runner-up first name in the middle if you plan on having more children. When parents do this, they usually think they'll want to start fresh and not recycle their old list when coming up with a name for a second child, or they're living in the moment and not thinking ahead. Both are perfectly reasonable ways to think about the issue, but now that I've come across so many parents who regret using their runner-up in the middle as they struggle to come up with a name for their second child, I recommend against it.

Other than that, my advice for middle names is simple: Either have fun with it or use it as a place to insert a meaningful name, but don't overthink it!

Putting It All Together: Name Flow

When thinking about the style and sound of a child's first name, there's one last thing to consider: How does it flow with the child's last name? Parents want their child to feel confident when they introduce themselves; they want a name that's cohesive and easy on the ears. But how do you achieve ideal name flow? There's no official rulebook about what makes a full name appealing, but a good rule of thumb is to say the name out loud and see how it rolls off the tongue. How is the rhythm? Do any sounds or syllables trip you up?

Often, parents with a last name that has harsh consonants want a softer-sounding first name to balance it out. If they have a long, complicated last name like Krzyzewski, they may want a straightforward and foolproof first name like Miles. Most people don't want the last syllable of the first name to be the same as the first syllable of the last name; a name like Arlo O'Brien is somewhat hard to say out loud. A first and last name that end with the same sound can be tricky too, as in a name like Brooks Hayes. And of course, if your child's last name is Graham, you may want to avoid the first name Teddy.

But at the end of the day, there are so many things to consider when it comes to a name that sometimes, you can't have it all. Think about your child's experience with their name. In most situations, people will address them by just their first name or by a title and last name (Ms. Jones, Dr. Smith)—not by their first and last name together, let alone by their first, middle, *and* last name. That's why my first priority is the first name, followed by the flow of the first name with the last name, then the flow of the middle name with the first name, then finally the flow of all three names said together (how often does that happen?!).

My last name is Slagen, and while I wouldn't name my daughter Reagan Slagen, I would consider naming a son James Slagen, despite the fact that the s's run into each other. I have a similar attitude when taking middle names into account: Lucy Maren Slagen doesn't sound as good as Lucy Marie Slagen, because of that repetitive -en sound, but if Maren was a family name I wanted to use to honor someone, I would definitely still go with it!

When you start to tune in to the naming world on social media, it can feel like name flow is critically important and you're committing a federal offense if you get it wrong. But for most people, including me, name flow is a consideration but not a top priority. I'm willing to sacrifice perfect flow if a first name checks all my other boxes. If name flow is one of the most important things for you, however, that probably helps you quickly narrow the field. And if you are willing to compromise on some elements, perhaps that opens up some names that you were not willing to consider before.

Make a list of your top first names paired with the child's last name. Say them out loud. Do they all pass the flow test?

_____

_____

_____

_____

_____

Make a list of your top first names paired with your top middle names. Which combinations are your favorite?

_____

_____

_____

_____

_____

Now combine your top first/middle name combinations with the child's last name. How do they look? How do they sound? Maybe your favorite first and middle names aren't part of your favorite combination, but they flow well enough. And that's perfectly okay!

Summarizing Style

I hope this chapter has helped you explore what you like and don't like about the styles of different names. And if this section made your head spin because you had never even considered half of these things, that's okay too! Everyone has different priorities and considerations in choosing a name. Highlight the elements that matter to you and leave behind the ones that don't. Remember that nothing is set in stone; these pages are valuable as a learning process even if you ultimately end up going in a totally different direction. Keep whatever lessons you learned in mind as you move to the next chapter, where we'll discuss another important aspect of the naming process: popularity.

· 3 ·

Popularity

The number one concern I hear from parents is: "I'm worried my favorite name is or will become too popular." For parents who were one of three Kaitlins or Megans or Emilys in their class growing up, they really want to avoid setting their child up for the same fate. But why?

For one, there's an inconvenience factor in having the same name as so many other peers or colleagues. You all turn your head at the same time. You get the wrong email. You constantly have to include the first initial of your last name to distinguish yourself. You get the wrong math test back and for a brief second panic that you didn't get an A.

Having grown up with a name that was familiar but not overly common (Colleen was ranked 159 the year I was born), I always found it to be a positive experience to meet someone else with my name. It was an instant way to connect, an assumed familiarity. But, strangely enough, in the Boston nursing world where I began my career, Colleen seemed to be as popular as Jessica or Ashley. In my relatively small division, I worked with two other Colleens, and I admit it did occasionally lead to confusion and miscommunications.

In large part, this concern is fueled by a general shift in baby name trends toward more unique names. This is a generation of namers who are less tied to tradition and are often looking for a name that feels fresh and uniquely "them." This is a generation of namers who celebrate diversity and individuality, who want their child to stand out rather than blend in. This is also a generation of namers who have access to baby name data.

As evidenced by Olivia's current longevity as a top 10 name for girls (since 2001!), many parents are not deterred by a name's popularity. A lot of these parents probably aren't even aware of the data and are simply choosing a name they've heard and liked (can you imagine such a straight-forward approach to baby naming?), while some parents may actually *like* that it's a popular name with universal appeal. Popular names also avoid the inconveniences that go with more unique names, like misspelling or mispronunciation.

Additionally, people can be drawn to more popular names because they're more likely to have neutral or positive associations with them, whereas with less common names, you might have only one association, and it might be negative. For example, if you've met a ton of Sarahs, the name Sarah probably doesn't remind you of anyone in particular, but if the sole Daphne you know of is the one from *Scooby-Doo*, you might be unable to get past the association and reject the name Daphne out of hand.

Fortunately, popularity is the one aspect of naming with some objectivity: We have data that you can use to help you make a decision. Let's dive in.

All other factors aside, if you could choose, how popular would you want your child's name to be? Circle one.

a) *If it ain't broke, don't fix it (in the top 100 names)*

b) *I want something that people have heard of but that isn't overly common (in the top 150–500 names)*

c) *I want something more unique (in the top 500–1,000 names)*

d) *I want something rare and unusual (outside the top 1,000 names)*

In some countries, certain unconventional baby names are actually illegal! In New Zealand in 2023, for example, the government registry rejected the names Prince, Princess, Messiah, Rogue, Sovereign, Captain, Chief, Empress, Pope, Notoriety, and Fanny.

Names by the Numbers

Every baby name consultant has one website bookmarked: the Social Security Administration (SSA) site on name popularity data. Every year, the SSA publishes a list of the top 1,000 most popular girl and boy names in the United States using the information submitted via applications for Social Security cards. For name nerds, the day this data gets released every year (usually in May) is like Christmas morning. It's not perfect; the SSA estimated that in 2023, their data represented roughly 71 percent of babies born that year (67 percent of female births and 75 percent of male births). But it is a great resource for understanding general baby name trends or a particular name's popularity.

The website is a name nerd's Disney World. You can search the top 1,000 baby names in any year going all the way back to 1879! You can find lists of the fastest-rising names and the names that are falling in popularity. You can find a list of the top 100 most popular boy and girl names in each state. (It's surprising how much this can vary from national data; for example, the name Juniper is ranked 113 nationally but 14 in Oregon!) You can search the top names of each decade or the top names cumulatively of the last 100 years.

My favorite feature is the ability to search an individual name and look at its popularity over time. It's fascinating to see the trajectory of a name like Luna, which wasn't even ranking in the top 1,000 until it came on the scene at 890 in 2003, but which skyrocketed to 10 in the most recent 2023 data! Or a name like Tessa that has demonstrated impressive consistency; since 1981, it's spent most of its time in the 200s. Or a name like Janet that spent 1928 through 1970 as a top 100 name yet hasn't even ranked in the top 1,000 since 2011.

The SSA data isn't limited to the top 1,000 names. You can download a separate file from the site that includes any name given to at least five babies that year. Some boy names used only five times in 2023 include Alby, Barlow, Barnaby, Daley, and McGuire. Some girl names used only five times include Alder, Babette, Crew, Evening, and yes, Beige. Though it's much more tedious to sift through than the top 1,000 list, it can be a great place to find unique baby name inspiration!

The United States has the biggest repository of name data, but there's data available in other countries as well. In many other English-speaking countries, you can find a list of the top 100 baby names. Australia, for example, does not have a national dataset, but you can find top 100 lists from individual states and territories. England, Ireland, and Norway are other examples of countries that publish the top 100 most popular names. If you're interested in a particular country, you can do a quick search to see what data is available, for popularity concerns or even just for inspiration.

Look at the number range you specified in the previous exercise. Look up the latest Social Security Administration data on SSA.gov and jot down any names in your desired range that appeal to you.

Name	SSA Rank

Breaking It Down

When a client asks me about a name's popularity, I like to put it in perspective. To show you what I mean, let's take a few different names as examples.

Say someone is considering the names Charlotte, Audrey, and Collins. In 2022, Charlotte was ranked number 3 in the US, Audrey number 67, and Collins number 247. This means there were about 12,891 Charlottes born (0.7% of total female births), 3,329 Audreys (0.19% of total female births), and 1,230 Collinses (0.07% of total female births). With the data representing about 2.6 million births in 2022 (of about 3.6 million total births), the difference between these numbers doesn't seem that impressive. And that's because, historically speaking, it's not. Compared to decades past, parents are using a greater variety of names, which means that today's popular names are being used with less frequency than the popular names of years past.

Let's take a look at the popularity of equivalent names in 1990. According to the website Our Baby Namer, the number 3 name, Brittany, was used 36,537 times, representing about 1.8% of female births that year. The number 67 name, Jacqueline, was used 5,238 times, representing about 0.26% of female births that year. The number 247 name, Mackenzie, was used 1,150 times, representing 0.06% of female births that year. As you can see, the number 3 and number 67 names each represented a larger percentage of births in 1990 than in 2022—meaning they were more popular than their modern equivalents with the same ranking. (The number 247 name was at about the same percentage.)

Let's rewind even further. Put on your poodle skirt and join me in the year 1955. The number 3 name, Linda, was used 51,288 times, representing about 2.6% of female births. The number 67 name, Julie, was used 6,786 times, representing about 0.34% of female births. The number 247 name, Ethel, was used 1,102 times, representing about 0.06% of female births. This means the number 3 and number 67 names were more common in 1955 than the equivalent-ranked names in 1990, which were more common than the equivalent-ranked names in 2022. (Once again, number 247 is at about the same percentage.)

Now, back to 2022. We've established that even the most popular names are more unique than the most popular names in decades past, but there are other factors to take into account as well. While Charlotte and Audrey have relatively similar rankings to the 2021 data (Charlotte ranked number 3 both years, while Audrey went from number 60 in 2021 to number 67 in

2022), Collins had a huge jump (number 328 in 2021 to number 247 in 2022). If you're leaning toward Collins, you might be wondering: Will it start to plateau next year, or will it continue to rise? Where will it peak? Anecdotally, I see Collins continuing to climb, as it's very on trend with the gender-neutral/surname style for girls right now, but I doubt it will become a top 25 name. Rapid growth can give a name a trendier feel, as compared to a name like Audrey that feels more classic and timeless, never ranking in the top 10 but never really going out of style either.

The data also gives us some (imperfect) insight into nicknames. If you do plan to use the name Charlotte, will you call her Charlotte, Charlie, or Lottie? While we don't know how many Charlottes go by a nickname, we can see that both Charlie and Lottie are on the rise right now as given names for girls, indicating their popularity. That being said, Lottie as a given name is ranked number 950, while Charlie as a given name is ranked number 123. So if you plan to use the given name Charlotte with the nickname Lottie, that's likely to feel much more uncommon than a Charlotte who goes by Charlotte or Charlie.

This may feel like a lot of math. What you probably really want to know is: Is there a meaningful difference in popularity between picking a name ranked number 1 vs. number 20 vs. number 100? The way a lot of people verbalize this concern is: "I love this very popular name, but I don't want my child to have the same name as three other children in their class."

For the most part, this is a much less common occurrence than it used to be, simply because of the diversification of names. However, while there may be only one Liam or one Olivia in your child's kindergarten class, those names have been popular enough for a long enough time that there will likely be at least one other Liam and Olivia in every single grade at the school, and you'll likely run into more Liams and Olivias at parks and museums and gymnastics classes.

In my opinion, if you're deciding between the number 1 name and the number 20 name, popularity shouldn't be a significant factor. Just go for the name you like more. If popularity is important to you, however, I think there's a pretty meaningful difference between the number 1 name and, say, the number 75 name—Autumn, as of this writing. While there may be only one Olivia and one Autumn in a given kindergarten class, there are more Olivias running around in general, so Autumn will feel like a much more unique name.

Regional Popularity

I have a confession to make: I cried the night after giving birth to my daughter. They were not tears of joy or tears of pain (those happened earlier). I was crying because I could not decide what to name her. If you're thinking that someone who'd been obsessed with names for thirty years would've had something picked out, that would be a fair assumption. But when the moment finally arrived, there were two names I loved so much I couldn't pick between them. After yelling at my husband for not giving me girl-girl twins and pleading with him to just write something on the birth certificate while I was in the bathroom, I—I mean, we—finally made a decision. We named our daughter Jane Reilly Slagen (both Jane and Reilly are family names, though I loved Janie before I knew that), and we call her Janie.

What was the other top contender that caused me so much anguish? Maeve. Maeve was a name I had liked ever since my friend told me she was babysitting for a little girl named Maeve when I was twenty-three. I have an affinity for Irish names, and I loved that I didn't know anyone with the name—but that started to change in the years around my daughter's birth. I was seeing it in articles about the hottest names and hearing it at every kid-friendly place I took my son. I worried that it would soon become too popular to align with my personal naming criteria.

And I was right.

Now you may look up Maeve on the list of most popular names in the United States in 2023 and think, *Number 75 is not exactly "too popular"* (and when I was naming my daughter in 2021, the most recent data I had showed it was ranked number 173). That's true—but *in Massachusetts*, where I live, Maeve is now at number 11. If I lived in California, where Maeve didn't even crack the top 100 in 2023, maybe I would've made a different decision about my daughter's name. But I encounter Maeves quite frequently where I live, and it just didn't feel special enough to me anymore.

My point is that if you're concerned with popularity, national name data tells only part of the story. And while we have name data for states, most of us can't look up data by city, town, or neighborhood. It could get even more granular: If your child goes to a Catholic school, you're probably coming across more Claires, Lukes, or other saint names than the average person. Regional and local trends may help explain why the data is telling you a name is quite popular yet you don't know any children with that name, or vice versa. At the end of the day, it's up to you to decide whether a name feels overused or unique *to you*, regardless of national rankings.

If you have any current top contenders, write them down here, then look up where they rank in the latest SSA data, both nationally and in your state. (If you think of other top contenders later, add them to the list.) Do they fall in the number range you chose in the previous exercise?

Name	SSA Rank (US)	SSA Rank (State)

The Social Media Effect

I had a client who loved the name Georgia but felt it was way too popular. She was surprised to learn it was ranked only 162 nationally (at the time) and wasn't in the top 100 in her state. She felt like she was seeing so many birth announcements on social media using the name Georgia. She was likely experiencing the social media effect.

We now live in a world where you know Brittany from your freshman dorm named her daughter Sylvie because you're "friends" via social media, despite the fact that you haven't spoken to her since college and she lives on the other side of the country. And you don't see the name Sylvie chosen just once—you see it over and over again on all the photos of name signs, chunky knit sweaters, and other baby paraphernalia she posts. Pair that with the rise of baby name content on various apps (guilty!), and you have the social media effect. It can make popular names feel even more popular, and uncommon names that you thought were uniquely yours start to feel taken or tainted.

Sometimes I post about a name style that's trending—like using surnames as given names for girls—and give examples of those types of names. People will comment things like "Nooo! Ellison is my girl name I've loved forever!" I try to reassure them that the name they love is still very uncommon—it simply falls within a name category that's trending and I happened to use it as an example. One name that epitomizes this phenomenon is Sloane. I've had so many clients list this as a name they like but won't use because it's too popular. It's actually ranked only number 151 as I write this, but I see it *all over* social media name lists and baby name paraphernalia, to the point that it's starting to make *me* wonder if it's going to jump to number 1 in next year's data.

Before you write off a name that really resonates with you because you think it's too popular, check the data and then look at names that have a similar ranking. Do *those* names feel popular? If not, you may be experiencing the social media effect, and you can feel free to choose the name you like without worrying.

Even in the 1700s, pop culture and news headlines were influencing baby names. In 1775, after reading a news story about General Richard Montgomery's death in a Revolutionary War battle, one patriotic American couple named their son Montgomery.

The *T* Word:
"Trendy"

There seems to be a lot of fear around picking an overly "trendy" name—a name that falls in and out of fashion super quickly. The fear here is less that too many of your kid's friends might have the same name and more that the name might feel time-stamped down the line: "Oh, that name is *so* 2025." I think the best way to avoid a time-stamped name is by looking at the data for the name you're considering and following the trajectory of its popularity over time.

On the boys' side, there are some obvious long-term heavy hitters like William, John, and Michael, but let's take a look at a slightly less obvious name like Simon. Since 1900, it has ranked between 198 and 552. This is quite a narrow range for a name over the course of more than a hundred years. It never falls completely out of fashion, yet it also never ranks among the top, trending names. This is the sign of a timeless name.

The equivalent is a bit harder to find on the girls' side, as there are more swings in popularity for girl names, but the name Caroline is a great example. Since 1900, Caroline has ranked between 55 and 329, another fairly narrow range. While Caroline has been a top 100 name since 1994, its ranking has remained relatively steady, never reaching inside the top 50. This still may be a more common name than you're looking for, but it's an example of a classic name that is unlikely to ever feel time-stamped.

A higher-ranked but still timeless example is Elizabeth, which, since 1900, has ranked between 6 and 26. An impressive feat! Part of its long-lasting appeal is its wealth of nicknames, which allow it to be flexible depending on current trends. Many years ago, Betsy and Betty were popular options, while Liz and Lizzie were more popular in the 1990s, and Ellie and

Ella are in line with current trends. Regardless, Elizabeth really stands the test of time and will likely continue to do so.

A name like Louise also feels pretty safe. It has had way more swings in popularity, ranging from as high as 17 to not even ranking in the top 1,000 in the 1990s and early 2000s. It finally started ranking again in 2016 and has been on a relatively slow uptrend since then. So, while you could definitely say it's on trend with the likes of other "vintage comeback" names, it's also an established name with a long history of use, giving it a classic feel, and it has ranked in the 600s for the past four years, making it much less likely that it will be as popular as other vintage revivals like Violet or Hazel.

What do you make of a name like Goldie, which ranks only at 685, but jumped about 200 spots over the past two years to get there? You also have to consider that Marigold ranks right alongside it at 714, and many Marigolds are nicknamed Goldie. While this does have the makings of a trendy name, I would still use it. Could it continue to climb and become a top 100, even top 50 name? It's possible. And perhaps if it were currently ranked in the top 50, I wouldn't use it, because if it was ranking that high, it likely would feel more popular and less special to me; I'd be more likely to know more Goldies.

Lastly, let's look at a name like Crew. This is a name that did not rank in the top 1,000 for boys prior to 2011. Since then, it has had a very rapid rise in popularity and currently sits at 260 (this does not account for the multiple other spellings that rank in the top 1,000). While it's not an overly popular name, it's newer on the scene and has had a rapid climb, which does indicate a trendiness. Sometimes the word *trendy* feels like the ultimate insult in baby name discussions, but it's not meant to be. A name like Crew is trendy because it's reflective of current cultural aesthetics and preferences. Because of its trajectory and its fragile roots, however, it's more likely to feel time-stamped or to fall out of fashion, compared to the steadfast Simon. At the same time, I don't think it's popular enough to date someone in the same way the name Linda (you were probably born in the 1950s) or Jennifer (you were probably born in the 1980s) would.

Keep in mind that you can also look at a list of names that are *declining* in popularity on the SSA website. While that can indicate a name is falling out of fashion, it can also be a sign a name has either found its spot or peaked.

If avoiding trendiness is a top priority for you, I would be most wary of names that are consistently having significant jumps in ranking—either rising or falling—year after year. But I want to assure you that it's okay to love a popular name, and there really are worse things than someone being able to guess the decade your child was born in from their name. And you can rest assured that because of name diversity, there will be fewer time-stamped names in this generation compared to generations past.

The Difference between *Trendy* and *Popular*

There's a difference between names that are *trendy* (they have a rapid climb and thus potentially a rapid fall from grace) and names that are perennially popular and currently *on trend*. The name Charlotte is very popular right now, but if you look at its popularity curve you can see that it's not truly trendy. It's a name that has been relevant since 1900. While it is having unprecedented success at the moment, it has always been common enough that I wouldn't worry it will feel dated or unfashionable down the line.

Compare this to a name like Everly. Everly had never ranked in the top 1,000 until 2012, when it skyrocketed to top 100 status. This reflected trends at the time: It started with an *E* and ended with -ly, and it was similar to another popular name, Evelyn. As of this writing, it appears to have peaked. It's starting to slowly fall in ranking and will likely continue to do so. I would describe Everly as trendy in a way that Charlotte is not (again, nothing wrong with a trendy name!).

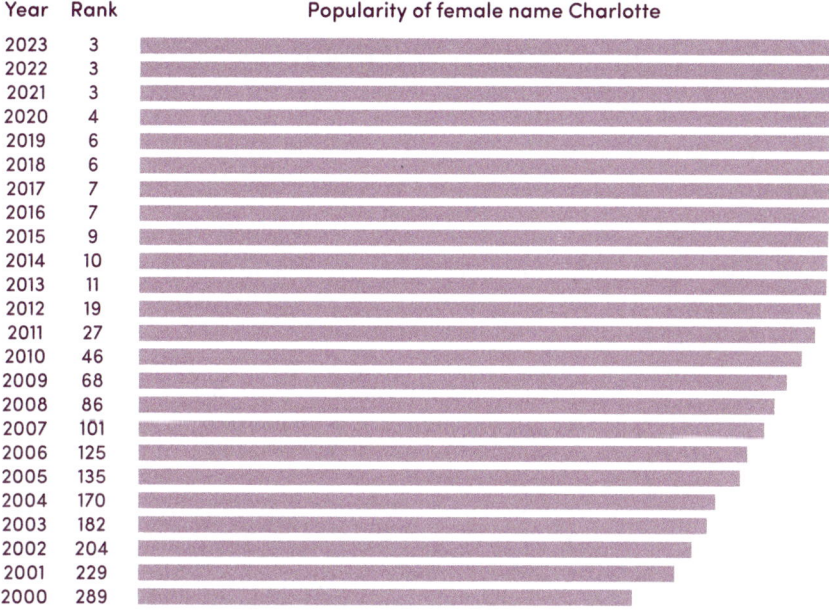

Year	Rank	Popularity of female name Charlotte
2023	3	
2022	3	
2021	3	
2020	4	
2019	6	
2018	6	
2017	7	
2016	7	
2015	9	
2014	10	
2013	11	
2012	19	
2011	27	
2010	46	
2009	68	
2008	86	
2007	101	
2006	125	
2005	135	
2004	170	
2003	182	
2002	204	
2001	229	
2000	289	

Source: Social Security Administration

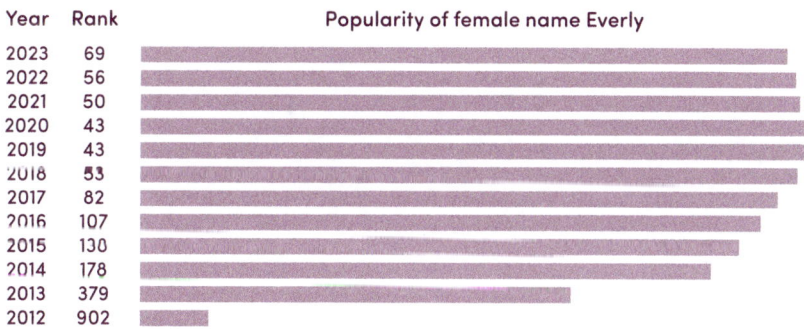

Year	Rank	Popularity of female name Everly
2023	69	
2022	56	
2021	50	
2020	43	
2019	43	
2018	53	
2017	82	
2016	107	
2015	130	
2014	178	
2013	379	
2012	902	

Source: Social Security Administration

On the boys' side, the name Luca is an example of an on-trend name that I think could attain classic status in time. While its popularity curve strongly resembles that of a trendy name—starting to rank in the top 1,000 only in the year 2000, with a fairly rapid climb to number 28—there is something unique about Luca. Although it didn't rank in America until 2000, it's a well-established name in other countries like Italy, so it doesn't feel like a new name the way Everly does. This is very similar to the name Liam, borrowed from Ireland and the UK. So, while Luca is definitely trendy, I think it will become more like Liam, a name that will likely stay in the top 100 for many years to come.

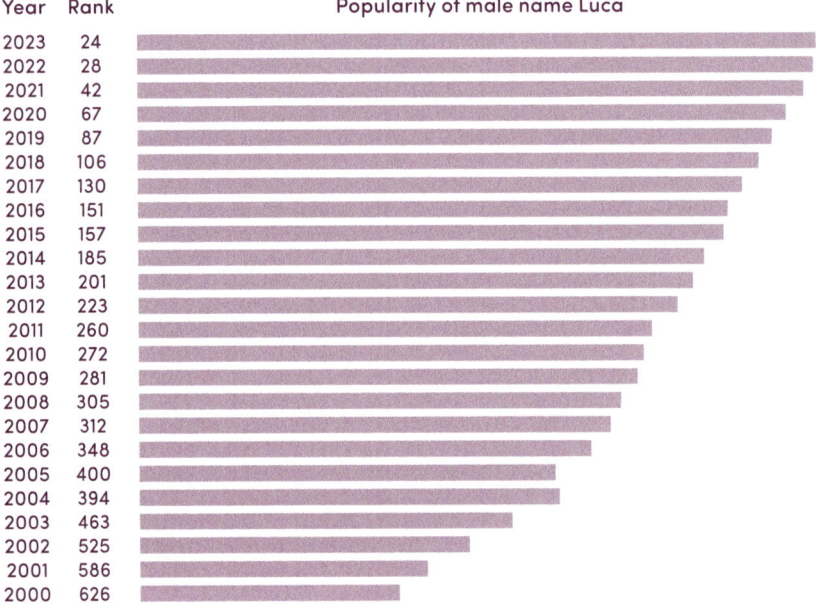

Year	Rank	Popularity of male name Luca
2023	24	
2022	28	
2021	42	
2020	67	
2019	87	
2018	106	
2017	130	
2016	151	
2015	157	
2014	185	
2013	201	
2012	223	
2011	260	
2010	272	
2009	281	
2008	305	
2007	312	
2006	348	
2005	400	
2004	394	
2003	463	
2002	525	
2001	586	
2000	626	

Source: Social Security Administration

This exercise will help you consider a name's popularity over time. If you have any current top contenders, write them down here, then search the data to see where they ranked in years past and how they rank today. Has their popularity gone up or down in recent years? Has the increase/decrease been fast or slow? (If there's been a very quick recent increase, the name might be considered trendy.)

Name	More/Less Popular?	Change Fast/Slow?

Names Inspired by Pop Culture

One aspect of name popularity that we can't always predict is pop culture influence; a name can skyrocket in popularity because a character in a movie or TV show has that name or because a celebrity chooses it for their child.

Luna got its first boost from the Harry Potter series and its second boost after Chrissy Teigen and John Legend used it for their daughter, which helped propel it to its current ranking of number 10. After the Jolie-Pitt twins, Knox and Vivienne, were born in 2008, Knox started ranking in the

Unpopular Names

In 1989, the year I was born, the SSA recorded that eleven baby girls were given the name Harper. In 2023, an estimated 7,769 babies were given the name Harper, making it the eleventh most popular name in America. Baby naming is one domain where making the unpopular choice can be appealing; perhaps you have the foresight to invest in a hidden gem. Most people who pick an uncommon name probably prefer it to stay that way, but there's something satisfying about being able to say, "I liked it before it was popular." Here are some of the names that were given to just eleven baby girls in the US in 2023: Aero, Anni, Apple, Artist, Axelle, Bri, Callum, Coast, Covey, Darcey, Damia, Dessie, Destin, Dori, Edison, Emiline, Erys, Ettie, Eulalie, Gabi, Galina, Giorgina, Grady, Grae, Holliday, Jeri, Lany, Lolani, Lotte, Lu, Lucette, Luxe, Makai, Perrie, Risa, Roxi, Sam, Steelie, Vali, Veya, and Zila. Thirty-five years from now, one of these names could replace Harper as number eleven.

top 1,000 in 2009 for the first time ever, and now ranks at 200; Vivienne has also experienced a rise since that year. In 2022, we saw several names from the show *Yellowstone* appear on the SSA's list of fastest-rising names, including Kayce, Tate, Walker, and Dutton. This not only reflects the popularity of the show but also aligns with the general trend of "modern cowboy" names currently having a moment.

A seal of approval from a celebrity isn't always a golden ticket to fame, though. Typically, to really succeed, a name has to be in line with a style that parents are already considering and can't be so unusual parents have never heard it before. Blake Lively and Ryan Reynolds used the name Betty for one of their daughters in 2019, and despite the fact that many vintage names are having a comeback, Betty has not ranked in the top 1,000 since 1996 (though it can be a nickname for Elizabeth, which the data does not account for). In addition, while many of the Kardashian baby names have risen in popularity since their use by the pop culture icons, many of them are too obscure to be widely adapted.

Here's a list of celebrity babies born recently who may influence trends over the next few years:

- Esti (Chrissy Teigen and John Legend)
- Adira (Serena Williams and Alexis Ohanian)
- Wren (Chrissy Teigen and John Legend)
- Rocky Thirteen (Kourtney Kardashian and Travis Barker)
- Aire (Kylie Jenner and Travis Scott)
- Ozzie (Mandy Moore and Taylor Goldsmith)
- Riot Rose (Rihanna and A$AP Rocky)
- Delphine (Joe Jonas and Sophie Turner)
- Bronze (Patrick and Brittany Mahomes)
- Cy (Jennifer Lawrence and Cooke Maroney)
- London (Paris Hilton and Carter Reum)
- Honey (Brody Jenner and Tiarah Blanco)
- Barrett (Bear) (Shawn Johnson and Andrew East)
- Townes (Hilary Duff and Matthew Koma)
- Caius Chai (Steph and Ayesha Curry)
- Denver (Jessie James Decker and Eric Decker)
- Krewe (Kane and Katelyn Jae Brown)
- Whimsy Lou (Nara and Lucky Blue Smith)

- Eloise (Sofia Richie and Elliot Grainge)
- Cardinal (Cameron Diaz and Benji Madden)

Sometimes people borrow a brand-new name from a piece of media, like Khaleesi from *Game of Thrones*. Khaleesi ranks 662, which isn't widespread but is much higher than I ever would have predicted. I had a client who was seriously considering the name Cersei, also from *Game of Thrones*. I have to admit, when I watched the first season of the show, that name really stood out to me for its soft, delicate sounds. That being said, I would probably steer away from it given this character's less-than-favorable arc.

The movie *Barbie* inevitably made its way into the baby name world a couple years ago, with many news sources asking baby name consultants if the movie would lead to a revival of the name Barbie. My answer: doubtful. A handful of parents might feel inspired to lead the vanguard of Barbara's comeback, but I think that's still a few decades away. I do, however, think the *Barbie* movie could have a major influence with a different name: Margot. Margot Robbie has a near-perfect public image, and the name possesses the elusive qualities that many parents are looking for in a girl name: timeless, feminine, versatile, and (previously) uncommon. Margot and its alternate spelling Margo have already started rising in the SSA data, and I would not be surprised to see them climb more in the coming years. On the other hand, one interesting psychological aspect of name trends is that now that we have access to data, parents react to it. If enough parents think Margot is going to become the next big thing, they may avoid using it, and it may not climb in popularity as much as the current buzz around the name would lead you to believe.

A pop culture reference can even have the opposite effect, causing a name to rapidly *fall* in popularity. You can see in the SSA data that Elsa had a big jump in 2014, as the movie inspired many parents to use the name. But soon the character Elsa was plastered on lunch boxes and clothing items in every minivan across America, giving the name a very typecast feel, and parents stopped using it. As of 2023, it no longer ranks in the top 1,000.

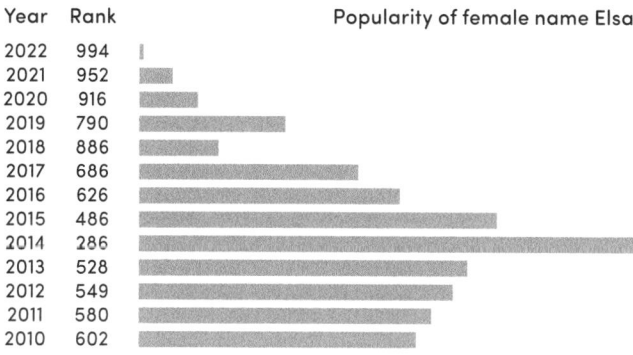

Year	Rank	Popularity of female name Elsa
2022	994	
2021	952	
2020	916	
2019	790	
2018	886	
2017	686	
2016	626	
2015	486	
2014	286	
2013	528	
2012	549	
2011	580	
2010	602	

Source: Social Security Administration

Unexpectedly Popular Names

Sometimes name trends seem to come out of nowhere—parents say they chose a name that no one else was using, but it ended up being a top baby name a few years later. This is an aspect of baby-naming trends that is perplexing and inexplicable even to name researchers.

To a certain degree, this is probably the exposure effect; things become more attractive to us with increased familiarity. So even though you may not personally have known any little Isabellas, you may have read the name in an article or a book or overheard it being used at the airport, without necessarily registering that you liked the name in that moment. You were exposed to it, you became familiar with it, you liked it. When this happens to enough people, it seems like everyone was thinking the same thing at the exact same time.

But the exposure effect cuts the other way too. If you become overexposed to something, you can get sick of it and stop liking it. That's why for some people, their top priority is to avoid having the next Karen or Emily or Jessica or Olivia.

In the end, you can study name trends, pore over the SSA's list of fastest-rising baby names, find the name with the steadiest popularity curve, maybe even pick a name from the list of names with the biggest drop in popularity from that year. But because of external variables like pop culture, no one can perfectly predict the trajectory of any given name.

How will you feel if you try to choose a unique name and it ends up being more popular than you expected?

_____

_____

_____

_____

_____

Client Consult:
Is Our Favorite Name Too Popular?

A pair of lovely clients came to me at the eleventh hour, six days before the mom's induction date, seeking a boy name to go with big brother Jack. They were looking for something that was well established but not overly common. Dad leaned more toward traditional names, while Mom was open to some more unique options. Their list included Henry, Theo, Brooks, Bennett, Luca, and Kyler, though Kyler and even Bennett felt like a stretch for Dad's taste. While they both loved Henry, they were worried about how popular it felt. Names they liked but couldn't use for various reasons included James, Callan, Logan, Canon, and Noah. Off-limits family names included Owen, Luke, Charlie, Emmett, Connor, Declan, and Pierce. Mom had vetoed Joseph, Nico, and Will, and Dad had vetoed Crew, Adler, and Graham.

Given the various styles across their respective lists, I wanted to include a variety of styles in their consultation, but I recognized that the classics seemed to be where they agreed most. I included classics like Teddy, Grant, and Elliott; some preppy vintage options like Beau, Wyatt, and Archie; surnames like Reid and Ellis; timeless but stylish options like Julian and Wesley; and some more modern Hail Marys like Penn, Gray, and Bowen. In their consultation, we also talked about how popular names are no longer used with the same frequency as the popular names of prior generations, so even a popular option like Henry or Theo wouldn't be as ubiquitous as popular options of years past.

The mom said she had read through an entire book of 100,000 baby names, *and* they had tried baby name apps, but hearing a fresh take on names they had skipped over, like Julian, gave them a new perspective that made it a top contender.

In the delivery room, it came down to Henry, Brooks, Wyatt, and Julian, then down to Henry and Julian. Finally, they ended up going with the handsome classic, Henry. For some parents, having popularity contextualized is very reassuring, as was the case here. There can also be something comforting about a more common name. You've heard it over and over and still find it appealing, as opposed to the risk of a new-to-you name like Julian, for which you worry your attraction could be fleeting.

We corresponded again months after the baby was born, and Mom expressed that the name Henry suited their son perfectly!

Are there names you've eliminated or vetoed because they felt too trendy or popular? Has reading this chapter changed your mind at all? Write down any names you may want to give second thought to now that you have some context on name popularity.

_____

_____

_____

Popularity in Review

We've now covered two of the most crucial elements of naming a baby: style and popularity. Whether or not you're a name nerd like me, you can use SSA data as a powerful tool to look up how popular a name is or just browse names for inspiration. (You can also flip to Part Two: Name Inspiration.) And if the idea of running searches and analyzing data numbs your mind but you really value understanding a name's popularity, that might be an indication that you'd benefit from hiring a name consultant!

Now that you've explored your thoughts and feelings on style and popularity, it's time to think about another very important element of naming a baby: family.

· 4 ·

Family Ties

A few years ago, when a friend of mine was pregnant, she had a discussion about baby names with her boyfriend's family. His mother had one firm suggestion: her own name, Aphrodite. (They did not land on this option.) Meanwhile, a friend of a friend planned to use Diane as her daughter's middle name, after *both* grandmothers—how fortuitous, right? Except one grandma spelled it Diane and the other spelled it Dianne, sparking a stressful and drawn-out debate of how to spell the name without offending someone.

Baby naming is an inherently familial process that connects a child to their parents and perhaps even past generations. That's beautiful! But it also means you might have to navigate boundaries with various relatives who want to influence what names you use or don't use. This chapter will help you consider what role you want family to play in your child's name— and give you a few creative ways to incorporate family names that may feel outdated.

Family Names

For a name consultant, getting your hands on a family tree is like uncovering precious fossils. Digging through your genealogical records for a name has many benefits. For one, it can help simplify your decision-making process, quickly narrowing down your pool of potential names from thousands to, hopefully, tens. It also gives your child's name a story, a rationale, something with a little more depth than "we just liked the name." If the namesake is living, it will undoubtedly be an honor for them, and if not, it gives the child a meaningful connection to their ancestry. I think this can be a great route to go, especially for people who really struggle with name indecision. It anchors your choice to something bigger than what could be a fleeting whim.

There are many different ways to incorporate a family name. Some people choose to pass down a family name for generations, creating juniors and thirds and so on. Others choose to honor a relative by using their first name and picking a unique middle name for their child, a balance between honoring family and giving your child their own identity. More and more, I'm seeing people get creative with family names: naming a girl Georgia after her grandpa George, or incorporating a family surname like Fletcher as a first or middle name.

The most common form I see is the use of a family name in the middle. This is usually the perfect compromise: If you want to pay tribute to a relative but don't totally love the name, stick it where it's a little less relevant. I am a big proponent of this. Is there a more beautiful or cohesive combination out there than, for example, Eloise Anne? Eh, probably. But if you're interested in honoring a family member named Anne, for me, that gets a trump card over first/middle name flow.

I had one couple who came to me with a unique challenge: Come up with a name for baby number four using the family tree they had acquired via a genealogy website. This baby would be joining siblings Edward (Ward), James, and Juniper (June), all of which were family names; Juniper was taken from the family name Geneva, which means "juniper tree." They had a girl name lined up but weren't connecting with any of the boy names they were seeing. My ideas for them included the following:

- **Cole:** based on the family name Nicolo
- **August/Gus:** based on the family surname Gustia
- **Fulton:** a family surname, with the nickname option Finn
- **Clarence:** a variant of the family name Clare, with the nickname option Clay
- **Rory:** a creative leap from the family name Roy, both of which mean "red king"
- **Reed:** based on the family surname Dozier, which means "from willow," referring to someone who lives near willows or reeds
- **Baker:** based on the family surname Semler, an occupational surname referring to a baker of white rolls
- **Taylor:** based on the family surname Snyder, which means "tailor" in German
- **Alder:** based on the family name Vernon, which means "alder grove"

After all that, they ended up with a little girl, whom they named Catherine Alice (both family names) with the nickname Kit—absolutely stunning! I found it so meaningful and impressive that they curated a beautiful set of sibling names using only honor names. What a fun consultation to be a part of!

Does the idea of using a family name appeal to you? Why or why not?

_____

_____

_____

_____

_____

If you're considering using a family name but haven't zeroed in on a specific one, write all the family names you can think of here, on both sides of the family, going as deep as possible. Consider aunts and uncles, great-grandparents, or even family members' middle names. If you want to, you can ask older relatives for the names of people who have passed on. If you have access to a family tree, you can consult that.

_____

_____

_____

_____

_____

Do any of the names you wrote above appeal to you? What about variations on any of them? Write them here.

_____

_____

_____

_____

_____

Reinventing a Family Name

Have you been tagged with the task of carrying out a family tradition and passing down a family name to the next generation? This is typically a tradition with fathers and sons, but it happens with mothers and daughters too. If you want to preserve the tradition but also give your child their own unique moniker, you can try adding a personal spin on the inherited name.

Let's say your child will be named John Daniel Miller Jr. To give him his own unique version of the name, you could use a nickname (like Jack or Jay), call him by his initials (JD), or address him by his middle name (Daniel, Dan, or Danny). If your child will be the third, fourth, or fifth generation with this name, a lot of these tricks may have already been taken, and you may have to get more creative!

Another route you can take is coming up with a nickname based on your child's numerical position in their sequence. Here are some ideas:

- **Second:** Chip ("chip off the old block"), Buddy, Sonny, Dub ("double"), Junior, add a J to their first initial (CJ = Christopher Junior)
- **Third:** Tripp ("triple"), Trey (slang for "third"), Trace (like the Spanish word *tres*), Bronze

- **Fourth:** Ivy or Iver (based on the Roman numeral IV), Four, Forrest, Ford, Dru (short for "quadruple"), Quade, Court (based on "quart")
- **Fifth:** Penn (like the prefix "penta-"), Quint, Quin, Quincy

If you've surpassed the fifth generation, I'm impressed by your family's dedication to tradition! Send me a message and we'll brainstorm!

Religious and Cultural Affiliations

Naming traditions vary across different cultures and religions, which can play a big part in naming a child. In Jewish tradition, you may choose a name that starts with the same letter as the name of a deceased relative. In Catholic tradition, parents typically incorporate a saint's name into either the first or middle name (see Saints' Names on page 176). Arabic names are often long, consisting of multiple family names following the given first name. In parts of Indian culture, horoscopes play a major role; the positions of constellations or planets at the time of the baby's birth are often taken into account when choosing the baby's name.

What I most often come across with my clients are parents looking for a name that feels modern and in line with their style but will easily translate when they're speaking another language or visiting family who speak another language. I also work with parents who want to give a name that honors their heritage in the middle slot while favoring a more American-sounding first name. I love the concept of continuing a religious or cultural tradition, and I think this can be a very grounding source of inspiration if you and your partner are struggling to come up with a name!

I once had the opportunity to work with a Chinese American couple looking to incorporate feng shui elements into their son's name. They knew this method of naming was new to me and fortunately gave me the opportunity to learn about it and work with them to come up with a unique, modern name for their son. The letters of the English alphabet were divided into columns that each had symbolic meanings, and my goal was to find a name that combined letters from each of the columns in a specific way. The names I recommended that fit the criteria included Decker, Denver, Xander, Vander, Calder, Rowan, Roman, and Murphy. It was both an honor and an exciting challenge for me to learn about a different style of naming and help come up with names that spanned two cultures!

Family Pressure

The reality of choosing a family name isn't always rosy. You may feel pressured to use a name you don't actually love. There may be competition between both sides of the family; if you're going to use only one family name, whose side will win out? Perhaps the people putting the pressure on you don't exactly feel namesake-worthy. (This is exactly why I could never join the royal family and give up all my baby-naming agency.)

Let me officially give you permission to forgo using a family name. To resist the urge to people-please. Don't get me wrong, I'm a huge proponent of incorporating family names and have used a family name in the first or middle slot for all of my children. But they should be used happily, not because of pressure and guilt. Naming a baby is a process that should be fun and supremely special. If considering family names is only adding stress to your life, then it may be time to reevaluate and move on.

This may be easier said than done, and everyone's situation is different. But the truth is, you can't always please everyone. Naming your Sims, your pets, your dolls is one thing, but this is the real thing. It's a uniquely personal experience and one you deserve to enjoy. So if you want to name your child Vesper instead of Laurence Cunningham Smith VI, by all means, you have my permission to do so!

Did you know Chip is an old-fashioned nickname for a junior or a boy named after his dad? It stems from "chip off the old block." This name has not ranked in the top 1,000 since 1978!

Compromising with Your Partner

There is one family member whose opinion you can't really ignore: your partner's. Finding a name that suits both partners' preferences is one of the most common dilemmas I see with clients: One partner likes classic names, and one partner likes more unique, modern names. One partner likes nicknames, and one partner is vehemently opposed. One partner wants to use a family name, but the other partner can't stomach it. Of course, not everyone naming a baby has a partner, but this section will offer some strategies for compromising for those who do.

This is a reality of baby naming that can feel like it takes the fun out of the process. I am a huge believer that this process can be enjoyable, from the debates over favorites to the discovery of a new contender. Try to think of it like a level 10 sudoku you're committed to solving rather than an impossible task that may result in marital tension and a nameless baby. Let's go through some strategies that I've seen work for couples who are at odds about baby names.

1. **Do your best to be open-minded.** While there are some names that are instant vetoes, sometimes we say no to a name simply because we aren't familiar with it. This can be especially true for couples where one partner is very passionate about baby names and spends a lot of time reading through name lists and discovering new ideas via social media. Familiarity breeds likeness. You may see the name Scout everywhere, but when you mention it to your partner, they say, "Scout?! Is that even a name?"

2. **Take it seriously.** Instead of having circuitous discussions at the dinner table, each partner should do a little research. There are so many great books, websites, and social media accounts out there that can open your mind to new ideas. Each partner should make a list in their phone and update it as they come across more names they like. Maybe it's really important for one partner to have a name of Hebrew origin. Look extensively at lists of Hebrew names. Can you get creative with any of them? Maybe there's a workable nickname you like for one of the names, or if you like gender-neutral names, maybe there's a Hebrew boy name that you love for a girl.

3. **Find the common ground.** Look at your respective lists. Is there anything they have in common? Perhaps even if your styles differ, you notice that you both like R names or you both tend to like boy names that end in o. If one partner likes gender-neutral names and

one likes feminine names, perhaps you can find a feminine name like Eleanor with a gender-neutral nickname like Leni. Narrow your name searches with the criteria you agree on.

4. **Compromise.** If it's getting down to the wire and neither partner is budging, you may have to decide whether to pick a "compromise name" that is neither partner's top choice but that both partners find to be suitable. Or if you plan to have more children, you could take turns so that each partner gets the final say from a list you agree on. I've had several clients who have gone this route, and ultimately both partners end up loving the name they landed on. (It helps when the name is associated with the newest love of your life!) I recommend making a call about how you plan to approach this *before* your newborn takes you to a new level of exhaustion.

5. **Get creative and have fun!** Make a PowerPoint presentation on why you think your partner should reconsider your favorite name. Include objective and subjective data as if this were a work deck. Maybe sprinkle in a few memes. Get access to your family tree for inspiration. Maybe surprise your partner with a video from a name consultant to lighten the mood and get some helpful tips or ideas. I recently had clients who ended up picking one of the boy names on my list of suggestions. The mom said she had suggested the name early on and it got rejected, but when I mentioned the name in the consultation with my rationale, it made her partner reconsider it in a new light.

I worked with one couple who could not agree on a name for their daughter, and it was creating a stressful baby-naming experience. Mom's taste leaned more vintage (Vivian), while Dad's leaned more traditional

(Madeline, Mary). They wanted something that would be cohesive with big sister Lucy, two to three syllables long, and outside the country's current top 10 names. A connection to a saint was also important to Dad. In their consultation, I suggested names that would bridge their individual tastes, like Florence (a feminine, vintage name that would allow them to use the family name Wren as a nickname, and a saint's name) and Colette (another saint's name that matches the elegance of Mom's favorite, but with softer sounds like some of Dad's favorites, plus lots of great nickname options like Lettie and Coco). Other names on their list included Caroline, Gemma, Cora, Iris, Cecilia, Eliza, Thea, Noelle, Molly, and Alice.

They ended up choosing the beautiful name Eliza Wren, which paired perfectly with big sister Lucy. They told me that having feedback, insight, and opinions from a neutral third party facilitated a much more fun and productive conversation about baby names—something to keep in mind if you're at an impasse!

What are some aspects of names you and your partner agree on? This could be anything: a general style, language of origin, religious affiliation, meaning, or specific letters or sounds.

_____

_____

_____

_____

If you and your partner disagree about a name because one of you thinks it's too unusual, try looking it up in the SSA data. It may be more popular than you think.

Name	SSA Rank

If you and your partner disagree on a name, try looking up creative nicknames for that name. Maybe you've always wanted to name your baby Margaret after your grandmother, but your partner vetoed it—but maybe they're agreeable to Daisy, which is a nickname for Margaret.

Name	Potential Nicknames

If you and your partner agree on a general style or aesthetic but can't quite agree on a specific name, try looking through Part Two: Name Inspiration. Do you see any names with a similar style that you might be able to agree on? If so, write them here.

_____

_____

_____

The Final Word on Family

Hopefully this chapter magically solved all your family disputes, and everyone now agrees that the name you suggested for this baby is without a doubt the best choice. If not, you probably made at least a little bit of progress or have some ideas for where to go next. If you still want to browse more names, see Part Two: Name Inspiration. And if you're facing other naming quandaries, don't worry. In the next chapter, I'll go through some of the most common naming conundrums I encounter in my work.

· 5 ·

Common Quandaries

We've covered a lot of territory so far: goals, style, popularity, and the role of family in naming a baby. But there are still a million little questions and hesitancies that can arise throughout the naming process. Will my kids' names look good together? If I have more than one kid, do I need to pick a theme for their names? Am I going to regret picking a unique name? Am I going to regret picking a common name? Is the name I choose going to affect whether my child gets their dream job? I looked through the many consultations I've done and polled my social media audience to compile some of the most common questions and worries parents have about baby naming. In this chapter, I'll try to address as many miscellaneous naming concerns as I can.

Naming Siblings

How do my kids' names sound when they're said together? How do they look together on holiday cards? What vibe do they convey? What assumptions might people have when they hear the names of our children? It's one of the most universal requests I get in consultation criteria: *We really want this name to complement our first child's name.* So let me share my personal philosophy around what makes sibling names cohesive as well as all the points you may want to consider when picking a name for a subsequent child.

As I've mentioned, I classify names into different aesthetic styles— "free spirit" names like Meadow and Ember or "modern cowboy" names like Ace and Colter. Most names are dynamic and could fit into several different style buckets. When thinking about sibling names that work well together, I visualize Venn diagrams of name styles that are cohesive with one another; for instance, classic names tend to pair well with vintage names and with surnames. For boys, August is a name that would be cohesive with other gentle-sounding boy names like Luca or Arlo, other vintage-sounding names like Hugo and Felix, or other nature-inspired names like Wilder or Alder. For girls, a name like Poppy can feel earthy and floral like Willow or Wren, posh and British like Beatrice or Camila, or snappy and cool like Liv or Maeve.

Aside from finding names that are stylistically cohesive, there are the phonetics to consider. Phonetics can be a way to tie together names that are stylistically different, but personally, I prefer names that are stylistically complementary rather than a phonetic match. So, while Liv and Maeve are stylistically cohesive, I would probably name two sisters Maeve and Blair or even Maeve and Willa to avoid using two one-syllable names ending in a *v* sound. However, this is not my top priority in choosing a name. If Maeve and Liv have been your favorite two girl names forever, the overlapping sound is not a deal-breaker in my opinion—and some people would argue that the final *v* sound actually makes them a great match.

I hesitate to get too granular, because I don't want to encourage overthinking, but, when naming a sibling, I also like to follow the three-letter rule: Sibling names cannot start or end in the same three letters. So Cameron and Camila, Hudson and Carson, and Adeline and Caroline would all be no-gos for me. If two names don't share three letters but do share a prominent sound, it depends on how common the sound is. Girl names that end in *a* are very common, for example, so Sophia and Lila work well together without sounding too matchy. For me, Elliot and Eloise are too similar, but Elliott and Bennett are okay. Roman and Rosie are too similar, but Rosie and Charlie are fine. Jane and James? Too similar. James and Brooks? That passes.

What about matching letters at the start of a name? In the baby name consulting world, most people say two is coincidence but three is a pattern. So, if you have Miller and Merritt, don't feel the need to choose an *M* name for your third child unless you love having a theme or are especially drawn to an *M* name. But if you have Miller, Merritt, and Marcie it starts to feel like that was on purpose. I hold a pretty liberal view on this; I don't think little Lane is going to be in therapy because his name didn't also start with an *M*. So if you're really stuck on coming up with a fourth *M* name, I wouldn't feel completely boxed in—but because there is a noticeable pattern at this point, I would be more inclined to lean into it. It's also easier to break a pattern when a pattern is already being broken: If you have three girls with *M* names and are pregnant with a boy, it feels more natural to choose a name with a different first letter. What you don't want is a situation where you feel so obligated to keep a pattern going that you name a child Jinger instead of Ginger to stick with a J theme (sorry, Duggars, but I have to call out a spelling error when I see it).

I once did a consultation for a family who unexpectedly found themselves with a C theme. These clients were searching for the perfect name for baby number four, a boy, who would be joining siblings Caterina, Cormac, and

Cole. (This is a perfect example of sibling names that come from different origins and have different styles yet work well together!) One of their biggest dilemmas was that they hadn't intentionally created this theme—their second child was going by Mac when they named their third child, so the alliteration was less obvious—and they weren't sure whether to continue it or to break the mold.

I didn't feel strongly that just because three kids' names follow a pattern, the fourth needed to follow suit. If it happened, great, but it wasn't something I would prioritize over choosing their favorite name. In their particular case, I did love how the letter C tied this unintentional sibling set together so well. I thought a great compromise would be to continue the trend in a more inconspicuous way by using a K name instead of a C name, using a soft-C name like Cyrus, or using a non-C given name with a C nickname like Pascal/Cal (or vice versa, like Carson/Sonny). My list of recommendations included Kieran, Callum, Joaquin, Hugo, Leon, Clark, Felix, Cedric, Ewan, Otto, Matias, Willem, and Simon, with several other C name options in the honorable mentions.

In the end, their older children really wanted to continue the theme, and they ended up choosing a wonderful name from their original list of top contenders: Conrad!

This is all fun to think about, but as I've mentioned before, it's up to you to decide how much priority it gets. Choosing the perfect name is not easy, and sometimes you have to be willing to give a little on some of your criteria in order to meet other, more important criteria. I will admit, when I was naming my first child we chose an Irish name that I had loved for a while. I wasn't really thinking about what I would name subsequent children— and I think most parents share a similar mindset when naming their first. Once I had him and was exposed to local baby names as I spent more time in child-centric circles, I realized how prevalent Irish names were in the

Sibling Sets

Here are ten examples of beautifully cohesive sibling sets that have stuck with me:

- Audrey, Rosalie, and Vera
- Esme, Florence, and Celine
- Ingrid, Perry, Dean, and Kit
- Clementine, Daisy, Juniper, and Autumn
- August, Oliver, and Daphne
- Lorelai, Gwendolyn, and Theodore (Lola, Gwen, and Theo)
- Rudy, Nell, Harriet, and Winston
- Silas, Gideon, Jonah, and Esti
- Vida, Iggy, and Teo
- Penny, George, June, Margot, and Ruby

Boston area and decided I didn't want to continue that theme with future children. While I still love his name, as a name aesthetic enthusiast, I do wish I had given more thought to the future sibling set (I leaned into more classic/vintage names for my next two children).

If sibling name cohesion is a priority for you, here are my top tips:

- Choose names that are stylistically, not phonetically cohesive. Use name websites or Part Two of this book to help you find name lists from specific categories.
- Stay away from names that sound too similar.
- Consider how many children you think you might have. If you do start a theme, is this something you'd want to continue for all of

your children? Will you feel limited in naming future children if you're beholden to a specific letter or syllable count?

How important is it to you that your kids' names complement one another? Circle one.

a) *This is a top priority for us.*

b) *It's a factor in our decision, but not the be-all and end-all.*

c) *It's not something we weigh heavily.*

What are the top five or so names you're currently considering? Write those alongside the name(s) of the child(ren) you already have. Say them out loud. How do they sound together?

_____

_____

_____

_____

_____

Naming Multiples

As baby name expert Sophie Kihm writes, "Naming twins is a rare opportunity to choose two related baby names at the same time that are compatible but also distinct."

I imagine it would be so deliciously fun to plan coordinating outfits, crib sheets, and baby accessories for multiples. It might be tempting to pick matchy names as well, but what we want here is peanut butter and jelly, not peanut butter and almond butter—names that feel complementary but not overly similar. I would avoid names that rhyme (Millie and Lily) or are the male and female versions of the same name (Emil and Emilia). A lot of people do lean in to matching first letters. While I personally would go with names with different first letters to minimize mix-ups, I admit it can work if the names overall have different sounds, like Edith and Eloise.

Aim for names with sounds that overlap without rhyming, like Hattie and Thatcher, Wallace and Louise, or Leighton and Gray. Or choose two names that don't necessarily sound similar but do fall into similar style buckets.

Classic	Vintage	Surnames	Nature-Inspired
Claire & Liam	Harvey & June	Quincy & Sterling	Willow & Sylvan
Madeline & Theodore	Dolly & Hugh	Riley & Quinn	Olive & Cypress
Jack & Elle	Sonny & Lottie	Calder & Merritt	Ivy & Jett
Margaret & William (Maggie & Will)	Pearl & Alfie	Murphy & Miller	Summer & Sage

Aside from sound and style, other ways to tie twin names together are through name origin (Kaia and Axel, both Scandinavian names), through theme (Stone and Bowie, both music-inspired), or through using honor names from your family tree.

There is also the question of who gets assigned which name. For some, it's easiest to approach it practically (baby A is Aveline and baby B is Elodie), but for some, it's important to meet the children to see which name fits which child better.

I worked with one couple who were looking to give their twin girls classic, feminine names that didn't feel too popular. They wanted the names to be short, easy to spell, and cohesive, with different starting letters. The names they brought to the table were Annie, Lily, Grace, Ellie, Emmy, Zoe, June, Nell, Mae, Hannah, and Jane. I added to the list Alice, Susie, Louise, Nora, Noelle, Rosie, Evie, Georgie, Ruby, Millie, Cate, Lottie, and Caroline. I incorporated all these names into the pairing suggestions, which included the following:

- Lily & Cate
- Lily & Caroline
- Jane & Lily
- Alice & Jane
- Gracie & Jane
- Annie & Jane

- Ellie & June
- Evie & Jane
- Alice & June
- Georgie & Louise
- Millie & June
- Nell & June

They ended up choosing the names Lily and Caroline, a beautifully classic combination!

If you're naming twins, do you plan to use a theme for both names? If so, what theme (same first letter, similar sound, similar style, etc.)?

_____

_____

_____

What are your top ten or so individual names? List them here.

_____

_____

_____

Now write down a few pairings from the list above. Circle any pairs
that go especially well together.

_____

_____

_____

_____

Different cultures have different approaches to the challenge of naming siblings. In Bali, children might be named based on their birth order, while in West Africa, they might be named based on the day of the week they were born.

Double-Barrel Names

Every once in a while, I work with a client looking for a "double-barrel" first
name like Mary Kate or John Paul. While these names are much more

prevalent in the South, you don't have to be Southern to see that combining two first names can make a traditional name feel fresh or serve as a way to tie in multiple family names. There's not much data on double-barrel names since most of them would be tallied in the SSA data by one name only (Mary for Mary Kate). Adding a hyphen (Mary-Kate) or removing the space between the two names (Sarabeth) can help ensure the second name doesn't get dropped. Double-barrel names are also more common for girls than for boys.

If you like the idea of a double-barrel first name or if it's a cultural or family tradition you want to uphold, here are some classic and more modern ideas for both boys and girls. I like the idea of combining something more traditional like Mary with something more modern or gender-neutral, perhaps a family surname like Mary Cameron, Mary Banks, or Mary Berkeley.

Classic (Girl)	*Modern (Girl)*
Lily Mae	Selah Grace
Clara Kate	Romee James
Emma Claire	Sasha Wren
Molly Mae	Lila Jaye
Daisy Jane	Della Dove
Anne Marie	Winter Mae
Jane Taylor	Poppy Jo
Ruby Rose	Maren Clare
Sadie Lee	Rowan Rayne
Millie June	Taylor Tate

Classic (Boy)	Modern (Boy)
Asher Luke	Beau James
Arthur Tate	Arlo Grey
Jack Michael	Luca Mays
John Henry	Grady Blake
John Hughes	August Lane
John Paul	Micah Jude
Miles Michael	Ziggy Roo
Noah James	Carter Cade
Simon John	Shepherd Shay
Thomas Mack	Hudson Hayes

Where to Find Inspiration

As a name nerd, I find so many names beautiful that the challenge is narrowing it down to only one. But some people have the opposite problem; they feel like they "just don't like any names." If that's the case, it's time to get inspired! Luckily, name inspiration is everywhere, from street signs to restaurant names to the brand of your favorite water bottle. I was in Warby Parker a few weeks ago and almost ran out of time to buy glasses because I was so distracted by the unique personal names they use as product names for each pair! I go out of my way to look for names in the wild: lingering a little too long at the swim class check-in to peep the other names on the attendance list, scanning every other coffee cup's label before grabbing my to-go iced latte at Starbucks.

The obvious name repositories are baby name books and websites, but the way names are typically presented there can leave you uninspired, with an empty list. You may skip over names that could be a really good fit because you're overwhelmed by the endless vault of random names in front of you. That's why I organized Part Two of this book by aesthetic style rather than alphabetically—so that if one name appeals to you, other names in the same style that will likely also appeal to you are right there on the same page. You could also use one of the Tinder-like name apps currently on the market (swipe left if you like a name, swipe right if you don't, find out which names you and your partner "match" on), but I will say, when I tried one, I found it pretty uninspiring, and my husband and I had no names in common.

If the usual sources aren't helping, it's time to start looking for names in more creative ways. I'll start by recommending a walk through a cemetery. It might sound morbid, but this is an especially great place to find some hidden vintage gems. If your tastes run more modern, another place to look is baby-product boutiques. Type "baby name signs" or "baby name sweaters" into a site like Etsy and you'll be inundated with (usually more on-trend) baby name ideas. Seeing a name next to an image of a real baby or seeing a first name paired with a middle name can give it a whole new feel!

And remember to be open because one positive association can completely change the way you perceive a name. There are plenty of names I like now that I was not as fond of a year or two ago. Hearing a name in the wild on an adorable child, hearing someone you admire say a name they like, hearing a name as part of a sibling set you like—experiences like these can change your perspective! If Jennifer Garner said she liked the name Bernard for a boy, it would likely become a new top contender for me.

If you're not interested in accessing your family tree for name inspiration, think of other ways you may find a meaningful name. Maybe you're from the West Coast and that's really important to you. Look up your home state's flower, the state bird, famous street names, or notable landmarks. Maybe you love literature; think about some of your favorite authors or characters for inspiration.

And don't forget to keep a running list and come back to it every so often. Names, like any other stylistic choice, can grow on you.

Name Regret

Most parents' worst fear when it comes to naming is that they'll regret their choice. One of the most surprising aspects of becoming a baby name consultant is how many requests I get to help parents decide whether to change their child's name, and if so, to what.

The other day, I was chatting with another mom who casually said about her daughter's name, "Yeah, I kind of regret that one." This is not the first time I've heard a sentence like that, but the difference between this nonchalant admission and true baby name regret is the pervasiveness of the feeling. As Kihm writes, parents in the latter camp "report negative feelings—such as anxiety, a pit in their stomach, or a sinking feeling—when they hear other people say their child's legal name. Often, these parents avoid saying their child's name aloud—they might use pet names like Baby or Buddy instead."

I've worked with several clients who were looking to change their child's name, from a few weeks to one year after the baby was born. The reasons parents regretted their initial name choice were varied. One client said she got a funny look from strangers when she told them her child's name. A few couples said they didn't know the gender going into delivery and hadn't put enough thought into names, leading them to make a spontaneous, rushed

Am I Overthinking It?

When you spend so much time thinking about a name, trivial concerns can start to feel insurmountable. I asked my followers for examples of this, and here were some of the responses:

- Does Maeve sound too much like my husband Dave?
- Is Campbell going to make people think of soup?
- Does Molly Jane sound like Mary Jane?
- Will my other daughter feel sad that her name is less unique?
- Are Jack, Teddy, and Caroline too Kennedy?
- Is it too presidential if I name my son Grant and my daughter Reagan?
- I wanted to use Arthur George but it's Rob Kardashian's sock line.
- Will my child struggle with possessives with a name that ends in *s*?
- Do Beck and Jack sound too similar for brothers?
- If I use James, will people call him Jim?
- Is it okay if my child has the initials MDD (major depressive disorder)?
- Do the initials NPD sound too much like NYPD?
- If my first baby's name starts with *A*, and I want to use a *B* name for this baby, am I going to have to use a *C* if we have a third?
- Is naming my son Tucker setting him up for a lifetime of bullying?

- If her last name will be Cooper, can I name my daughter Minnie?

You don't need to make sure the first letters of your children's names follow the alphabet, NPD does not make me think of NYPD, and I had no idea Rob Kardashian had a sock line, but I would avoid the name Minnie if your child's last name is Cooper. If you're preoccupied with a concern like this, run it by some trusted friends to get a sense of whether it's valid or you're completely overthinking it!

choice, especially with the pressure the hospital put on them. One client who picked a more uncommon name was feeling bad after negative reactions from family; another picked a common name without realizing how popular it was. A few clients felt like they conceded to a name they never liked to please a partner. One chose her favorite name despite her hesitation about how it sounded with their last name, only to regret that choice after saying it out loud more once the baby had arrived.

Some of these clients came to me having doubts, unsure of what to do. In those cases, I first tried to understand what wasn't working with the current name and then explored if there was a way to troubleshoot it. Other clients came to me having already made a firm decision to change their child's name and wanting some help this time around. Some of these clients went on to change their child's name, and some ended up sticking with their original choice. (One ended up feeling better about her original choice after working with her therapist.)

The decision to change your child's name is extremely personal, but be aware that you may feel even more pressure to get it right than you did during the first go-around, making it even harder to select a name. Every situation is different and for some people, a name change is the fix, but for others, there may not be any name that feels satisfactory. If the anxiety is all-consuming, it may be worth talking to a therapist. If you want to discuss some of your holdups with a name or how to work with the name you chose, or if you've decided to proceed with a name change, that's when a baby name consultant would be helpful.

I want to assure you that it *is* okay to change your child's name instead of letting it eat at you for the rest of your life. For the clients I have worked with who decided to go through with a name change, despite an agonizing decision-making process, in the end they reported feeling great relief. But at the same time, if you're having feelings of name regret, know that you are not alone and it doesn't always warrant a name change. Even if your child's name doesn't feel perfect at the moment, they'll make it their own in due time.

Here are some tips to help you avoid or cope with name regret:

- Don't go into the delivery room unprepared. Have a list ready with the top two to three names you've agreed on.
- If you really struggle with naming one specific gender, it may be worth finding out the gender instead of going into the delivery room without a name ready.
- If you're really unsure about a name, tell at least one or two trusted family members or friends who will give you honest, reasonable feedback.
- Make sure you say the full name you plan to use out loud. When I

was deciding on a name for my daughter, I had my two-year-old say our top contenders to test them out.

- If you're experiencing baby name regret, act sooner rather than later. The longer you wait, the harder it will be mentally.
- Think about ways you could work with the name you chose: nicknames, middle names, initials, and so on.
- If you follow baby name accounts, it may be a good idea to unfollow them after your baby is born.

Name Claiming

The only thing worse than someone stealing your grocery cart when you were 95 percent done with your shopping is someone "stealing" your coveted baby name. When someone uses your favorite name, it can be a huge disappointment. There are various iterations of this type of tragedy, which range from completely innocent to downright egregious. The most flagrant variety ("I told my sister-in-law my favorite girl name was Mila and she said she'd never considered it, but then she used the name Mila") is pretty rare. It's much more likely that someone in your family or friend group shares the same taste as you and thus landed on the same relatively common name.

What's the best strategy for dealing with name "stealing"? Do you keep your top choice in Fort Knox in the hopes that no one uses it before you, or do you proclaim it to family, friends, neighbors, coworkers, and the bank teller in an effort to stake your claim? Let's talk through name-claiming etiquette. There are several factors to consider that would affect how I would approach different scenarios.

Who's Using the Name?

The first thing to consider is who wants to use the name. If your sibling or sibling-in-law uses a name before you do, that pretty much rules it out for me (although this can be very normal in certain cultures). What I do think is okay is using names that sound similar, like using Eleanor even if your brother used Eloise.

If it's your cousin or another relative outside your nuclear family, it's a little more complicated. How often do you see them? Do you live in the same town and hang out all the time, or do you see them only every so often for weddings and funerals? If it's the latter, while most people still prefer to avoid names already used in their family, I think it's okay to repeat if it's the name you've had your heart set on or if it's a family name. You and your cousin whom you rarely see both want to name your sons after Grandpa Leo? Go for it! If it were me, I would probably have a quick conversation about it just to avoid ruffling feathers.

If it's your coworker who already used the name, or a girl from high school you follow on social media, or someone else who isn't part of your inner circle, then use it! I get that a name can feel "used" or no longer novel if you find out someone else claimed it, but with modern-day connectedness, you're often going to be able to find someone else who's used a name.

How Common Is the Name?

The second thing to consider when someone else has claimed a name you like is how common that name is. The more popular the name, the less hesitant I would feel to use it. Think about how many people in the same neighborhood or social group have had kids named John at the same time.

Now, if the name you wanted to use was Liora and a close friend already used it, I would be more hesitant, because it's so distinctive. That being said, this is a personal choice. If someone else using it taints it for you, grieve the loss and move on; there are lots of great names out there! If you still want to use the name but don't want to be seen as a copycat or name thief, it's worth having a conversation with the person. If you picked out the name Liora when you were fifteen and you can't let go of it, I think most friends would be reasonable about that. There is nothing wrong with two people having the same name!

How Reasonable Is the Person?

Another factor to think about is whether the person who already claimed your name is generally reasonable and able to resolve conflicts. If one of my friends wanted to use one of my kids' names, even if it were someone I see fairly often, I would feel more flattered than offended. It's entirely possible that your friend or relative will feel the same way. If you think they'd be up for it, it's worth having a light conversation. Of course, you have to be aware that they may say no, so if you're going to use the name regardless, think about how you want to word the conversation. Do you want to politely ask for their blessing to use the name, or do you want to inform them in a friendly way that you'll be using the name as well?

What If It's an Animal, Not a Person?

Is it okay to use a name if someone you know is already using it for their pet? I'm only half joking here. I've had several people come to me asking if they can use their favorite name if it's already the name of their mother-in-law's dog. My first question is usually "How old is the dog?" After that, my second question is "How stuck are you with names?" I have so many girl names I love that if my sibling or parents had a dog with one of those girl names, I would just rule it out and move to the next one on the list. My boy list is much shorter, though, so if I had one favorite boy name, I would consider still using it (especially if it was also a family name—in one case, someone told me she wanted to use Theodore/Teddy after her grandfather, but her in-laws had a dog named Teddy).

What If *You're* the "Thief"?

You know your best friend has always loved the name Birdie. But you love it too, and it turns out you married a guy whose beloved grandmother was named Birdie. You're both pregnant with girls, but you're due a month earlier. Solve for *x*.

I know some people feel more territorial than others about names, but I am not that person. I would have a conversation with the person, with the outlook of "How fun would it be if our daughters had the same name!" You also have to take the particulars into account. In this example, if it weren't for the family connection, I'd say to forget about Birdie and find another name. But if it feels like *the* perfect name that both you and your partner agree on *and* it has a meaningful family connection, I think it's a conversation worth having. My opinion here changes if it's a sibling or sibling-in-law who has already said they want to use Birdie. In that case, it's time to look elsewhere.

Someone I Know Chose a Name I Hate

If your friend, family member, or even a random mom at the park announces their child's name and you hate it, it's okay to lie. Don't give some obviously backhanded reply like "Where'd you come up with that?" Don't make a face. If someone asks you for honest feedback prior to naming their child, that's different. But once they've chosen a name, there is no reason to say anything other than "Great choice" or "That's so 'you guys' it's perfect." It doesn't mean you aren't genuine; it means you're rising above your impulse to give your opinion when it's not welcome. You can imagine the pressure I feel when someone announces their child's name to me. If I don't comment on the name, that's a statement! I can always find something positive to say, even if it's not a name I would choose. The last thing a postpartum mom needs to hear is that you don't like her precious baby's name; save those comments for your text thread with your best friend.

Will My Baby's Name Determine Their Future?

It's natural to wonder what impact the name you choose will have on your child's life. Will certain names set them up for career success or doom them to an unhappy future? Nominative determinism is the idea that people are drawn to careers or interests that align with their names—a chef with the last name Cook, a geologist named Rocky, a wealthy businessman named Richie.

Beyond these entertaining associations, some studies have concluded that people with easier-to-pronounce names are more likely to have higher-status positions, that women with gender-neutral names are more likely to succeed in male-dominated fields, and that people with stereotypically white-sounding names are more likely to get job interviews than those with names that sound Black. But there are also studies that come to different conclusions, and it's difficult to believe that other factors (like the unfortunate realities of sexism and racism) aren't playing a much bigger role than name choice. And any of these effects could become outdated as cultural trends shift.

Beyond social inequities, is Westford more likely to be a CEO or doctor than, say, Blossom? It's possible that the types of parents who favor a name like Westford are doing other things that put their child on a path toward a high-powered career, as compared to parents who choose a more hippie name like Blossom. But there is no data to support a causative link between name aesthetic and career. While a name may influence micro-outcomes, there are so many more complex aspects of both genetics and environment that will impact a child's future.

Perhaps a more realistic question to ask is "Will my child like their name?" But even then, you can't predict the future. Maybe they'll find it annoying that they always had to correct people on spelling or pronunciation, or maybe they'll love that they always stood out. Maybe they'll lament that their name was so common, or maybe they'll enjoy having some anonymity when people try to Google their name. And more than likely, their opinion on their name will change during different phases of their life. They may not like how much their unique name stands out during those insecure years in middle and high school, but as an adult, they may really embrace it.

The bottom line is that your child's future will not be made or ruined by their name. Hopefully that eases a little bit of pressure!

Concluding Common Questions

I hope this chapter has helped solve some of the common naming dilemmas you might be facing, provided you with ideas for name inspiration, and given you some strategies to address some of the more complex challenges like name regret. Some people choose to keep baby names completely private until the big reveal, but I always think it's helpful to have one or two trusted friends with whom you can discuss your naming questions and worries. Now it's time to wrap things up and talk about how to settle on that one perfect name.

· 6 ·

Choose a Name

Throughout this book, we've covered more aspects of baby naming than you probably thought possible. When you began reading, you likely had some sort of baby name challenge, which this book hopefully helped you out with. Maybe you had no names you liked, and now you have ideas of where to look for inspiration. Maybe you and your partner couldn't agree, and now you have some strategies for compromising. Maybe you had concerns about popularity, and now you have some context that helps you make a decision. Now we've arrived at the final chapter, and it's time to put it all together and choose a name!

Arriving at Your Name

Some couples will have a light bulb moment where one partner discovers a name that the other partner instantly takes to. But more than likely, it'll be a little less climactic and after tireless discussions, you'll say something like,

"So we're good with Hazel Greer then?" Some people have their child's name picked out ten years before conception, some people have the aha moment while they're pregnant, and some people are still debating the name while the nurse waiting to fill out the birth certificate gives them raised eyebrows on day three of their hospital stay.

Personally, I'm a mix of the first and the last. To no one's surprise, I've been thinking about names forever and have always had a running list. The problem is I love discussing names so much that I don't actually want to settle on a name before the last possible minute! I'm more of a practical namer than an intuitive one, so I don't go into labor thinking that when I see the baby, all of a sudden the right name is going to hit me (but many people do have that experience!). For this reason, I like to come to the delivery room prepared but open. I usually have a top contender with one or two fierce competitors I'm keeping on reserve.

Either way, pick the approach that best suits you and your partner. If naming has been really difficult for you, don't count on the idea that seeing the baby is going to make things suddenly click. I can tell you from experience the postpartum hormones don't do you any favors when it comes to decision-making!

This exercise won't be for everyone, but if you're a Type A, spreadsheet-loving kind of person, try out this ranking system for your top contenders and see which one scores highest. First, assign each of these categories a percentage in terms of how much they matter to you. If a category doesn't matter to you at all, give it a zero. All the percentages should add up to a total of 100.

Popularity: _____%
Ease of pronunciation: _____%

Sibling cohesion: _____%

Name flow: _____%

Meaning: _____%

Gut feeling: _____%

Now write your top contenders in the table below and rate them on a scale of 1 to 5 in each category.

- **Popularity:** 1 indicates the name is very unique and 5 indicates it's very popular.
- **Ease of pronunciation:** 1 is very difficult to pronounce and 5 is very easy to pronounce.
- **Sibling cohesion:** 1 is not cohesive and 5 is very cohesive.
- **Name flow:** 1 indicates poor flow and 5 indicates great flow.
- **Meaning:** 1 means you don't like the meaning and 5 means you love the meaning.
- **Gut feeling:** 1 means no gut feeling and 5 means a strong feeling keeps pulling you back to this name.

Name	Popularity	Pronunciation	Sibling Cohesion	Name Flow	Meaning	Gut Feeling

Now use this formula to calculate a score for each name:

[Popularity score × Popularity %] + [Pronunciation score × Pronunciation %] + [Sibling cohesion score × Sibling cohesion %] + [Name flow score × Name flow %] + [Meaning score × Meaning %] + [Gut feeling score × Gut feeling %] = _____

Name	Score

Which name has the highest score?

_____

What Really Matters

Between family and friends and especially social media, there's a lot of outside noise these days when it comes to choosing a baby name. At the end of the day, the most important thing is that the people having the baby love the name. Here are some final pieces of advice:

- **Try not to get too caught up in popularity.** Be aware, but don't overstress. If finding a name that isn't popular is a top priority

When to Call the Professionals

If you still can't choose a name, here are a few reasons to call in backup and hire a professional baby name consultant.

- You need someone with the time and expertise to do a deep dive into name meanings and family trees.
- You and your partner have opposing naming styles, and you need a third party to find something you can both agree on.
- You're not planning on discussing names with family and friends and want an objective professional to weigh in.
- Just for fun! Of course you don't *need* to pay someone to help you name your child—you also don't *need* to splurge on a designer stroller or an organic French teething ring, but sometimes you do it anyway! And unlike a teething ring, a name will last forever.

for you, great, you know that immediately eliminates the top 20 names (or top 50, or whatever your line is). But if you love a popular name, that's okay! Remember that popular names are used with less frequency nowadays, and there are many benefits to having a popular name. Your child's life will not be ruined because they had another Evelyn in their class!

- **Do your due diligence.** Do a basic name "screen." Look at what the initials would be, say the name out loud in its entirety, think through potential nicknames, look at the name meaning, and say it with any siblings' names. This should help you catch any flagrant faux pas.

- You're naming a person, not a baby. It can be tempting to picture the names on your list only on an adorable little baby, but remember the baby stage is temporary. So if you like a name that perhaps feels a little formal for a baby, don't worry, they'll quickly grow into it!

- Think beyond the name announcement. This is where a lot of your insecurities about picking a name may play out in your head. *People are going to think I copied someone. People are going to say those names don't sound good together. People are going to think it's too weird. People are going to make fun of the middle name we chose.* The name announcement is a brief moment where it feels like you're presenting your baby's name for the world to judge. Yes, you should be proud of your baby's name. But remember that after the announcement, your baby's full name will not be the subject of constant scrutiny.

- Know yourself. Are you someone who will be devastated if someone makes a negative comment about the name you chose? Or can you quickly flip the script and say, "Wow, they're rude." This mostly goes for people picking a more unique name. If you're not prepared to own it and brush off negative feedback, it may be worth running it by a trusted friend or objective third party for reactions.

- Have fun with it and follow your gut! What's the name you'll be sad to let go of? When you tell people the names you're considering, what name do you hope they'll call out as their favorite? When you hear the name mentioned by someone else you think, *Hey, that's our name.* Trust your instincts and know that the overthinking will be a distant memory once your precious little baby embodies the name.

Here it is: the final exercise!

Write down your top five names.

Boy	Girl

Write down your top two names.

Boy	Girl

Write down your baby's name!

Boy	Girl

In Conclusion

As a society, we're completely fascinated by baby names. If you're pregnant, the second question you get after "Do you know if you're having a boy or a girl?" is "Do you have a name picked out?" Once you have the baby, people politely utter the obligatory "Is everyone healthy?" before chomping at the bit to find out the baby's name. News outlets compete to be the first to announce a celebrity baby name. Name announcement posts on social media get huge clicks. Even people who are not pregnant or don't plan to have children can't help but read articles about the top baby names, muse with a friend about what names they would choose, or discuss the latest provocative celebrity name. My ninety-five-year-old grandmother, Mimi, can't remember that I've lived in Boston for the past ten years or that she already asked me two minutes ago if I wanted coffee, but she remembers the names of all my children.

I always thought I was an outlier with my lifelong obsession, but the internet has magnified a collective infatuation that has always existed. What is it about names that fascinates us? In the same way we obsess over fashion choices at award shows or analyze the details of someone's home renovation, we think about baby names as a style choice—but with bigger stakes.

Naming a baby is a form of self-expression we bestow on another person, a glimpse into whether we prefer to conform or stand out, a conscious or unconscious message about our values and priorities. It's a coalescence of our curiosities, imaginations, and egos (and, sometimes, our worst impulses to judge others). Although naming your child is personal and meaningful, on a surface level, names are a form of pop culture and a way for us to assert our worldviews. When you delve deeper into a name, it can speak to issues like gender, religion, race, socioeconomic status, history, family, and even the subjective personality traits you associate with a certain name.

It's easy and fun to contemplate names, casually dissecting the latest baby name announcement on your social media feed in your group chat, discussing baby names with the pregnant mom next to you on the airplane, or guessing what the royal family will name their newest baby. But when it's your turn to take the stage, the benign daydreaming can suddenly transform into a pressure cooker of anxieties, fears, and overanalysis.

If I told you names are not a big deal, it would be like a dentist saying you really don't *need* to brush your teeth every day. So I won't say that exactly. But what is critical to remember is that even though this is one of the first decisions you make as a parent, there are way more important decisions you'll make that have a meaningful impact on your child's life. So while, yes, you should put thought into your child's name, remember that a lot of the stress is social pressure you can safely ignore, and that baby names can be one of the most fun aspects of pregnancy.

If you've officially settled on a name, congratulations! I know that this will be the perfect fit for your little one, and if it's possible, your fondness for this name will grow even more once they're here. If you haven't settled on a name yet, what I hope you've gained from this book is not just insight, ideas, and objective strategies for approaching the baby-naming process, but also a restored or newfound joy in the process. We get to do this only so many times, so we may as well have some fun with it. Rest assured that whatever name you choose, your child will infuse it with meaning and character and personality as they grow. Best of luck finishing your name journey, and maybe I'll see you back here for the next one!

name inspiration

You've arrived at Part Two of the book, which is packed with thousands of potential names to use as inspiration on your own naming journey. But instead of organizing them in one big alphabetical list, I've grouped them according to aesthetic style. That way, instead of getting lost in a sea of unrelated names, most of which won't appeal to you, you can consider names in similar categories. Names are dynamic, so you'll find some names that fit into several different categories. If you like a rugged name like Nash or Maverick, the Modern Cowboy list will provide other names in the same vein. If you favor a name like Daisy or Marigold, the Garden Glam list will help you out with other floral names. Feel free to dog-ear, bookmark, and take notes in the margins—and most of all, enjoy!

Biblical

If you want a traditional biblical name, you probably don't need a name consultant, as there's a very big book that has all the information you could possibly need. Still, these tried-and-true names are worth mentioning because they've stuck around for a reason. They're as great today as they were two thousand years ago. **See also:** Biblical (Bible Chic), Saints' Names, Traditional (with Nicknames).

GIRLS

Abigail	Lydia
Anna	Magdalene
Bethany	Mara
Claudia	Martha
Deborah	Mary
Delilah	Miriam
Dinah	Moriah
Elizabeth	Naomi
Esther	Noemi
Eve	Phoebe
Hannah	Rachel
Jemima	Rebecca
Joanna	Ruth
Judith	Sarah
Julia	Susanna
Leah	Tabitha

BOYS

Aaron	Asher
Abraham	Benjamin
Andrew	Caleb

Daniel	Joseph
David	Joshua
Elijah	Luke
Ethan	Mark
Ezra	Matthew
Gabriel	Nathaniel
Isaac	Noah
Isaiah	Paul
Jacob	Peter
James	Philip
Jeremiah	Samuel
Joel	Simon
John	Zachariah

Biblical (Bible Chic)

If the traditional-feeling biblical names are too plain for you, but you're still looking for a name with a connection to the Bible, you may want something in the style I've fondly nicknamed "Bible chic." These are names that appear in the Bible or other Judeo-Christian texts but may be names of places rather than people (Bethlehem) or are simply less common than your Matthews and Marks. A lot of these names have risen quickly to popularity (Silas, Levi, Eden), while many still remain quite uncommon (Gideon, Junia, Selah). This is a great place to look for a traditional, established name with a more contemporary or edgy feel. **See also:** Biblical, Saints' Names.

GIRLS

Adah	Mercy
Adina	Mikiah
Apphia	Myra
Ariel	Noa
Atara	Priscilla
Bethlehem	Rhoda
Beulah	Salome
Clementia	Sapphira
Cleo (from Cleopas)	Selah
Eden	Shiloh
Eliora	Shoshana
Emmanuella	Surah
Eunice	Talitha
Helah	Tamar
Jael	Zipporah
Junia	

Abner

Amos

Asa

Barnaby

Bartholomew

Boaz

Cain

Cyrus

Ezekiel

Felix

Gideon

Jericho

Jesse

Jonah

Jonas

Judah

Jude

Levi

Malachi

Matthias

Micah

Moses

Phineas

Reuben

Roman

Samson

Shiloh

Silas

Solomon

Titus

Tobias

Zaccai

Zeb

Zion

Zuriel

Boomer Names, Refreshed

While many of the most popular names of the 1950s and 1960s feel outdated and likely won't be making a comeback anytime soon, baby boomers are in their grandparent era, and their children may want to try to honor their parents' names, but with a modern twist. For example, maybe your mom's name is Linda; you could use Linden as a middle name for your daughter. Or maybe your dad's name is Ronald; you could use Veronica as a first or middle name. Or if you're looking to go against the grain, be the first to bring one back, like Meghan Trainor did when she named her son Barry Bruce. The names here offer a refreshed spin on popular boomer names. I've grouped them into "Girls" and "Boys" based on the original boomer name, but you'll find suggestions for masculine and feminine "refreshed" names in both lists. **See also:** Millennial.

GIRLS

Amy: Ames, Bellamy

Ann: Annette, Annie, Annelise, Susanna, Grace (Ann means "grace")

Beverly: Everly, Ever, Evie

Brenda: Brennan, Brendan, Brenn

Carol: Caroline

Cynthia: Thia/Thea

Darlene: Lena, Darling

Eileen: Eilee, Lena, Birdie (Eileen means "little bird")

Elaine: Elle, Laine, Lainey

Ellen: Leni, Eleanor, Elle, Nell

Helen: Helena, Nell, Leni, Lena

Janet: Jane, Jay, Etta

Joan: Jo, Joey

Judy: Judah, Jude

Julie: Juliet, Jules, Julien

Karen: Wren/Ren, Karys

Kathleen: Kate, Kit

Laura: Laure, Laurel, Lauren

Linda: Linn, Linney, Linden

Lisa: Lisette, Elise, Lise

Lois: Lo, Loey, Louis

Margaret: Daisy, Maisie, Margot, Rett

Nancy: Cy
Patricia: Cia, Patrice, Reese
Sandra: Andi

Susan: Susanna, Lily
(Susan means "lily of the valley")
Teresa: Tessa, Tess, Teres, Reese

BOYS

Anthony: Ant, Tonie
Carl: Carlie, Carlisle
Charles: Cal, Caroline, Charlie,
Charlize, Charlotte
Clarence: Clara, Clare, Ren
Dale: Daley
David: Davie, Davis
Dennis: Arden, Dennie
Edward: Teddy, Ward
Eric: Erickson, Errol
Frank: Frankie, Franklin, Frances,
Francis, Francesca
Gary: Garrison, Gray
Gregory: Rory

Jeffrey: Rey, Reya
Joseph: Josephine, Effie
Kenneth: Kennedy
Lawrence: Law, Rencie, Ren
Leonard: Leo, Lenny, Leni
Mark: Marcel, Marcelline
Michael: Mick, Mac
Phil: Philippa, Pippa
Robert: Bo, Bobbie
Scott: Scottie, Scottlyn
Stephen: Stevie
William: Liam, Wiley, Billy

Boy Names for Girls

Giving a conventionally male name to your daughter is a way to use a traditional name in an unexpected and unique way. Some parents feel that using a boy name for their daughter will serve her well in a world that often favors men. Historically, as a name becomes more popular for girls, it starts dropping in popularity for boys, but as more and more names start being used for both genders and people become more open to the idea of names being fluid, that pattern may start to dissipate. Most of the names listed here don't even rank in the top 1,000 for girls, but Logan, Noah, and Elliott are increasingly mainstream. Some parents choose to feminize the spelling, like changing Elliott to "Elliette" or Everett to "Everette." **See also:** Feminine Names with Gender-Neutral Nicknames, Gender-Neutral, Masculine/Gender-Neutral Names with Feminine Nicknames, My Best Friend's Dad.

Asher	Callan	Everett	Levi	Sawyer
August	Carlisle	Ezra	Logan	Smith
Austin	Chandler	Gray	Luca	Spencer
Beau	Clarke	Harvey	Madden	Sterling
Beckett	Colby	Hunter	Mason	Stewart
Beckham	Conner	James	Max	Toby
Bennett	Davis	Jett	Miles	Tyler
Bevan	Declan	Johnie	Murphy	Wallace
Bradley	Drew	Jude	Noah	Wells
Brady	Dylan	Kyle	Owen	Wesley
Brooks	Easton	Landon	Pierce	Wilder
Bryce	Elliott	Lawson	Randall	Wiley
Callahan	Evan	Leo	Ryan	Wyatt

Celestial

Science nerds meet horoscope enthusiasts. Do you want to give your child a name that is mysterious and otherworldly? Look no further than celestial names, which reflect a sense of wonder and beauty in the world. While some of these have become among the most popular names in America (Aurora, Luna, and Leo), many remain rare gems for parents looking for a distinctive baby name with a connection to nature. **See also:** Greek Mythology, Nature-Inspired, Outdoorsy, Roman Mythology.

GIRLS

Aster	Juno	Seren
Aurora	Jupiter	Skye
Calliope	Luna	Soleil
Caprice	Lyra	Star (Starry, Starlie)
Celeste	Meridian	Stella
Ciel	Moon	Sunny
Estelle	Nova	Vega
Halo	Selene	Vesper

BOYS

Apollo	Elio	Oberon
Aries	Galileo	Orion
Atlas	Leo	Phoenix
Comet	Major	Sirius
Cosmo	Mars	Triton
Draco	Mercury	Zephyr

Cool Girl Names

These ladies can talk their way out of any ticket and convince you to go to Yacht Week two weeks before your nursing boards exam. There is something effortlessly chic about one-syllable girl names. Liv Tyler, Blythe Danner, Storm Reid; they all wear it well. One-syllable names appeal to parents who want something light and no-nonsense. This generation of parents feel less tied to giving their child a formal name just for the sake of formality; thus the appeal of a lot of one-syllable nicknames as given names. She's Liv, not Olivia. She's Bea, not Beatrice. Short, two-syllable names hold a similarly stylish appeal. Many rank in the top 100, like Isla, Eden, and Lyla, while some rank outside the top 1,000 like Alba, Gaia, and Ines. There is something inherently cool about this category of short and chic girl names. **See also:** Edgy Boy Names, Gender-Neutral, Modern Cowboy/Cowgirl, Short and Sweet.

ONE-SYLLABLE

Bea	Eve	Love	Sage
Belle	Gray	Lux	Sam
Bette	Greer	Maeve	Scout
Bex	Gwen	Neale	Shay
Blair	Hope	Nelle	Skye
Blake	Jade	Neve	Sloane
Blythe	Jones	Nyx	Storm
Bree	Jules	Paige	Teale
Bryce	Kai	Pearl	Tess
Bryn	Kit	Pip	True
Dove	Lake	Quinn	Wren
Drew	Laure	Rain	Wynn
Elle	Liv	Rome	Wythe

Alba	Ines	Nina
Alta	Isla	Nori
Ara	Juno	Petra
Ayla	Lana	Remi
Caia	Lela	Rhea
Cleo	Lena	Rio
Davy	Lovi	Romi
Demi	Luna	Roxy
Eden	Lyla	Suki
Ella	Mari	Suri
Esme	Mia	Tova
Esra	Mika	Vada
Esti	Mira	Vera
Ever	Nara	Zara
Gaia	Navy	Zoey
Indi	Naya	Zuri

Cottagecore

Do you aspire to raise your kids on a homestead, perfecting your sourdough starter and effortlessly teaching them math by measuring flour and sugar? Or maybe you live in New York City and buy your organic milk for $7.99, but *if things were different*, you'd be putting on the wool cardigan you knitted by the fire to go grab some fresh milk from your family cow. This is the trendy concept of cottagecore, which glamorizes a homesteading existence. Even if you'd prefer to get your groceries via Instacart, you might find names with this aesthetic charming! **See also:** Cozy by the Fire, Old Hollywood, Vintage Darlings, Vintage Grandma and Grandpa.

GIRLS

Alice	Mabel
Betty	Maisie
Bonnie	Marjorie
Cordelia	Marnie
Dorothy	Martha
Esther	Millie
Etta	Nell
Felicity	Polly
Fern	Posie
Florence	Prudence/Prue
Frances	Rosalie
Greta	Sally
Harriet	Sylvie
Josephine	Wilhelmina
Lottie	Winnie

Albie	George
Alfie	Gus
Ambrose	Hank
Archie	Harvey
Augustine	Huck
Benedict	Hugh
Charles	Leonard
Earl	Lewis
Edwin	Percy
Ernest	Reggie
Eugene	Sonny
Franklin	Thatcher
Gene	Winston

Cozy by the Fire

Some names have the power to create a sensory experience, evoking vivid imagery like the smell of freshly picked flowers on a spring afternoon or the sound of crashing waves during a summer storm. Of course, it's all subjective, but for me, this list of names feels warm and cozy, like you're sprawled across a leather armchair with a knit blanket, reading a book by the warmth of a crackling fire with a glimpse of a snowy winter landscape out the window. **See also:** Cottagecore, Old Hollywood.

GIRLS

Abigail	Fern	Madeline
Adeline	Flora	Marjorie
Alma	Freya	Martha
Annora	Greta	Miriam
Aurelia	Gwen	Noelle
Autumn	Harriet	Polly
Aveline	Hazel	Rachael
Beth	Imogen	Rosemary
Blythe	Iris	Ruth
Briony	Jane	Scarlett
Cornelia	Joan	Sonora
Cosima	Josephine	Sylvie
Edith	Laurel	Tamsin
Eleanor	Lenore	Tess
Esther	Linnea	Wendy
Felice	Luella	Wilma

Arthur	Ezra	Monty
Asher	Fitz	Oliver
Auden	Florian	Oscar
Auggie	Gabriel	Owen
Benjamin	Graham	Penn
Bernard	Grover	Remy
Cassius	Harold	Robin
Cecil	Heath	Rudy
Charlie	Joseph	Sam
Cyrus	Julian	Shepherd
David	Laurie	Sonny
Ernest	Linden	Wilder
Errol	Loren	Will

Edgy Boy Names

Edgy boy names are contemporary and unconventional. They feel strong, confident, and maybe even a touch rebellious. A little bit trendy, a little bit bold, these names appeal to the parent looking for a distinctive name with a modern aesthetic. I could easily mistake this list for the starting lineup of a college baseball team. Even as toddlers, these guys probably dress better than you do. **See also:** Cool Girl Names, Modern Cowboy/Cowgirl, Surnames as First Names.

Ace	Dax	Keir	Rhone
Baird	Dex	Kemp	Rhys
Banks	Drake	Knox	Ridge
Beau	Duke	Lex	Riv
Beck(s)	Fitz	Link	Rome
Blaise	Fox	Locke	Rune
Bond	Gage	Mack	Slate
Bray	Guy	Mav	Steele
Brigg	Hart	Mills	Stone
Cade	Hawk	Nash	Tate
Camp	Hayes	Pax	Teague
Cash	Hux	Payne	Ty
Chance	Jax	Penn	Van
Chase	Jay	Price	Vance
Cole	Jett	Rafe	Vaughn
Crew(s)	Jones	Reeve	Wes
Cruz	Kai	Rex	West
Dane	Kane	Rez	Wolf
Dash	Keane	Rhodes	Zane

Axel	Iver	Phoenix
Bauer	Jensen	Radnor
Bishop	Lando	Rainer
Bode	Ledger	Ramsey
Bridger	Lennox	Rigby
Camden	Levi	Roan
Dyer	Luca	Ryder
Fletcher	Milo	Ryker
Hardy	Myer	Slater
Harley	Onyx	Viggo
Hendrix	Oslo	Zander

Feminine Names with Gender-Neutral Nicknames

If you can't decide between a more feminine name and a more gender-neutral name for your daughter, don't worry—this is a situation where you can have your cake and eat it too by choosing a traditionally female name that easily nicknames to something more gender-neutral. Versatility is the name of the game. **See also:** Boy Names for Girls, Gender-Neutral, Masculine/Gender-Neutral Names with Feminine Nicknames, My Best Friend's Dad.

Addison: Sonny

Alberta: Albie, Bertie

Alexandra: Andie

Ariel: Ari

Augusta: Gussie

Aurora: Rory

Bernadette: Bernie

Camila/Camille: Cam

Cecily: Cy

Charlize: Charlie

Cordelia: Corrie

Edith: Eddy

Eleanor: Leni

Elizabeth: Eli

Elowyn: Wynn

Francesca: Frankie

Georgia: Georgie

Geraldine: Geri

Harriet: Harrie

Henrietta: Henrie

Jacqueline: Jack

Josephine: Joey

Judith: Jude

Juliet: Jett

Kennedy: Kenny

Leona: Leo

Loretta: Rett

Louisa: Lou

Mackenzie: Mack

Margaret: Garet

Martha: Matty

Matilda: Matty

Maxine: Max

McKenna: Mack, Kenny

Michaela: Mickie

Nicolette: Nic

Olivia: Ollie

Ophelia: Opie

Penelope: Penn

Peregrine: Perrie

Persephone: Percy

Philomena: Phil

Prudence: Denny

Rebecca: Beck

Regina: Reggie

Robin: Robbie

Samantha: Sam

Scarlett: Scottie

Stephanie: Stevie

Sydney: Syd

Teresa: Reese

Theodora: Theo

Veronica: Ronnie

Victoria: Vick

Wilhelmina: Will, Billie

Winifred: Freddie

Free Spirit

If you embrace the idea of your child having a unique name, crave the response "I've never heard that before" when you introduce your child, or long for a family of boho adventurers, "free spirit" names have you covered. Some of these names are trendy, some are invented, but they all give off a cool and creative aesthetic of little tots running wild and free along the beach while you pitch the family tent. **See also:** Garden Glam, Influencer Names, Outdoorsy.

GIRLS

Arlie	Ever	Lovie	Sol
Aura	Fable	Maeva	Sonnet
Autumn	Florie	Meadow	Star
Belvie	Haven	Norie	Story
Bindi	Honey	Novi	Sunny
Birdie	Indie	Ottie	Tiggy
Bliss	Isley	Peace	True
Bloom	Ismay	Peachy	Twila
Blue	Jewel	Peri	Valley
Cova	Journey	Petal	Velzy
December	Jovie	Pixie	Vesper
Dovie	Juniper	Prairie	Willow
Echo	Juno	Primrose	Winslie
Elkie	Lemon	Rain	Winter
Ember	Leni	Romie	Zeah
Essence	Lilou	Rue	Zori

Aero	Fox	Sage
Aspen	Harlow	Sky
Banjo	Jordy	Sonny
Banksy	Koa	Sparrow
Bear	Koda	Tide
Bleu	Lucky	Valen
Bodhi	Marley	Van
Bondi	Oakley	Wave
Bowie	Obi	Wilder
Cove	Odie	Wolf
Dune	Reef	Zepp
Dusk	River	Ziggy

French

If you read *Bringing Up Bébé*, you know there is something appealing about French parenting—and French names. These names will undoubtedly breed a precocious toddler who can negotiate bedtime with the charisma of a seasoned lawyer, sniff out the finest cheese at the tender age of three, and win the prize for "best dressed" at every playground. French names, especially French girl names, are on the rise in America. Regardless of whether you come from French-speaking roots, these names drip with elegance and sophistication. Names like Margot, Sylvie, and Josephine are now mainstream, and less common options like Soleil, Amelie, and Elodie are potential up-and-comers. For boys, Remy and Hugo are in the top 300, with Lucien and Florian on the rise. **See also:** Quiet Luxury, Romantic.

GIRLS

Adele	Brigitte	Elodie	Lilou	Perrine
Adelie	Camelia	Eloïse	Lisette	Raphaelle
Alix	Camille	Emilie	Louise	Rosalie
Amandine	Capucine	Esme	Lucienne	Sabine
Amelie	Cecile	Fleur	Madeleine	Simone
Anaïs	Celeste	Genevieve	Manon	Soleil
Appoline	Celine	Georgette	Marceline	Solène
Arlette	Cerise	Helene	Margaux	Sophie
Armelle	Chloe	Ines	Marguerite	Sylvie
Aurelie	Claudette	Josephine	Marie	Therese
Avril	Clementine	Julienne	Marlene	Violette
Azelie	Colette	Juliette	Nathalie	Vivienne
Babette	Cosette	Justine	Nicolette	Zelie
Beatrice	Delphine	Laure	Noelle	
Bijou	Elise	Leonie	Odette	

Alain	Gabriel	Mael
Alexandre	Gael	Marcel
Andre	Gage	Mathieu
Antoine	Gaston	Noel
Augustin	Gerard	Olivier
Beau	Guy	Pascal
Bertrand	Henri	Pierre
Blaise	Hugo	Quentin
Claude	Jacques	Raphaël
Clement	Jean	Remy
Corentin	Jules	Rene
Dax (place-name)	Julien	Sebastien
Emile	Laurent	Sidney
Etienne	Lebron	Valentin
Fabien	Louis	Xavier
Florian	Luc	Yves
Francois	Lucien	

Garden Glam

Floral and plant-inspired names for girls are never out of style, but they can take on a variety of aesthetics. We have mainstream classics like Lily and Rose alongside vintage cuties like Daisy, Iris, and Marigold, which have a sprinkle of hippie whimsy but could also belong to little girls in big bows and white linen dresses. And of course there are the full-on flower-child names like Saffron, Willow, and Clover that evoke a carefree, one-with-nature existence. This list of girl names feels like a bright summer day! **See also:** Free Spirit, Nature-Inspired, Outdoorsy.

Acacia	Flora	Marigold
Azalea	Ginger	Peony
Blossom	Holly	Petal
Bluebell	Hyacinth	Poppy
Briony	Iris	Primrose
Calla	Ivy	Rose
Camellia	Jasmine	Rue
Clementine	Jessamine	Saffron
Clover	Lavender	Sage
Dahlia	Lilac	Senna
Daffodil	Lily	Violet
Daisy	Linnea	Willow
Fern	Magnolia	Wisteria
Fleur	Maple	Zinnia

Gender-Neutral

Versatile and flexible, gender-neutral names are growing in popularity. As the trend gains traction, I expect people will feel even more confident and attracted to the idea of bending gender norms in the naming world. All the names listed here can, by definition, be used for any gender, but I've divided them into girl-leaning (used more often for girls) and boy-leaning (used more often for boys) based on the 2022 SSA data. **See also:** Boy Names for Girls, Cool Girl Names, Surnames as First Names, Feminine Names with Gender-Neutral Nicknames, Masculine/Gender-Neutral Names with Feminine Nicknames, My Best Friend's Dad.

GIRL-LEANING

Aspen	Emery	Leighton	Quinn	Skylar
Avery	Finley	Lennon	Reese	Sloane
Blair	Frances	London	Remi	Sunny
Blake	Greer	Marley	Riley	Sutton
Briar	Harlow	Marlowe	Sage	Tatum
Eden	Harper	Oakley	Shay/Shea	Taylor
Emerson	Hollis	Palmer	Shiloh	Wren

BOY-LEANING

Alex	Carter	Francis	Layton	River
Ari	Casey	Hayden	Lennox	Robin
Baker	Chandler	Hunter	Logan	Rory
Baylor	Drew	Jamie	Madden	Rowan
Camden	Dylan	Jordan	Noah	Sawyer
Cameron	Elliot	Kai	Parker	Sonny
Carson	Ellis	Lane	Remy	Spencer

Globe-Trotter

Whether it's your hometown (mine is Vienna, Virginia!), where you went to college (Charlottesville), or a memorable place you've travelled (Annecy in France comes to mind), place-inspired names have a lot to offer. They can evoke a sense of natural beauty, worldliness, or connection. They may be reflective of a specific culture or landscape that carries a certain aesthetic. For example, the name Capri feels chic and sophisticated, while Montana feels rugged and outdoorsy. Choosing a globe-trotter name can be a way for parents to express their values or aspirations and add a personal touch or distinctiveness to their child's name. This is a list of less common place-inspired names.

GIRLS

Alaska	Dakota	Italia	Milan	Sedona	Vail
Annecy	English	Lexington	Montana	Seneca	Valencia
Arizona	Florence	Lille	Olympia	Seville	Verona
Aspen	Geneva	Lisbon	Paris	Sicily	Vienna
Avalon	Georgia	London	Quincy	Sonoma/	
Bali	Havana	Louisiana	Ravenna	Sonny	
Cambria	Holland	Lyon	Roma	Sorrento	
Capri	Indiana	Malta	Salem	Tulsa	
Carolina	Ireland	Marseilles	Scotland	Tuscany	

BOYS

Auckland	Caspian	Everest	Nile	Rhodes	York
Boston	Chicago	Houston	Oslo	Rio	Zealand
Brighton	Copeland	Hudson	Palermo	Rome	
Brisbane	Cypress	Israel	Phoenix	Rouen	
Bronx	Denver	Kingston	Raleigh	Sheffield	
Cairo	Durham	Nashville	Reading	Tex	

Greek Mythology

Names from Greek mythology serve as a unique source of inspiration for the modern parent with a penchant for history or literature (or astrology or even video games). While they have a unique and colorful feel, these names are deeply rooted in tradition and, for the most part, familiar. Names from mythology often have symbolic meaning, cultural connections, or an association to nature or the cosmos. **See also:** Celestial, More to Love, Roman Mythology, Romantic.

GIRLS

Artemis	Clio	Maia
Asteria	Cyrene	Nyx
Athena	Daphne	Penelope
Aura	Delia	Persephone
Bronte	Echo	Phoebe
Calliope	Electra	Selene
Charis	Gaia	Thalia
Chloe	Hera	Xanthe
Circe	Iris	

BOYS

Achilles	Hector	Sirius
Adonis	Jason	Titan
Apollo	Leander	Troy
Atlas	Orion	Zephyr
Cadmus	Paris	Zeus
Damon	Perseus	
Eros	Pollux	

Influencer Names

As with celebrities, the baby names chosen by social media influencers often feel heavily unique, ahead of the trend (their virality probably starts the trend in a lot of cases), and even provocative, resulting in polarized opinions from their audiences. One family who turned heads with their name choices are the Funks, an influencer couple with 1.6 million followers on Instagram and 2.4 million on TikTok who named their children Super, Sweetie, and Storm. Some of the names listed here are the actual names of influencers' babies, while others are just in line with that style. Influencer names push the limits of current naming trends and guarantee something memorable and unconventional. **See also:** Free Spirit, Unique.

GIRLS

Apple	Echo	Lyric	Soul
Aspyn	Evening	November	Spirit
Baby	Ever	Peach	Spring
Bambi	Fig	Pebble	Star
Bear	Gal	Pepper	Story
Blondie	Halo	Poet	Sugar
Blue	Heart	Rebel	Sunday
Busy	Hero	Reverie	Sweetie
Cricket	Honey	Romance	Theory
Cozy	Honor	Rumor	Trixie
Darling	Island	Scout	True
Dear	Lore	Sonnet	Wednesday
Dreamy	Love	Sosa	Whimsy

Alfa	Elvis	Ranger
Anthem	Four	Reef
Blues	Fox	Rocket
Brave	Hawk	Seven
Breeze	Hennessy	Smokey
Cape	Huxley	Space
Cash	Knight	Stoic
Champion	Legend	Super
Chaplain	Lion	Tiger
Chief	Major	Valor
Cosmo	Million	Wisdom
Cross	Noble	Writer
Cruz	Phoenix	Zealand
Edge	Pilot	Zion

Irish

Irish names have the benefit of feeling classic and established, yet modern and fresh. Most of the names we think of as Irish are really anglicized spellings, like Declan for Deaglan or Maeve for Maebh, as parents may be hesitant to bestow a name that is likely to get frequently misspelled and mispronounced in America. The flipside is that native Irish names will often be a conversation starter and represent pride in your Irish heritage. (To that end, I've included both anglicized and non-anglicized versions on this list.) Additionally, using Irish surnames like Reilly, Murphy, or Callahan as given names is a popular and stylish take on incorporating your heritage. And at a time when gender-neutral names are very appealing to parents, Irish names like Rowan, Finley, and Rory work well.

GIRLS

Aileen	Dara	Lennon
Ailís/Ailish (AY-lish)	Darby	Maeve
Aine (ON-ya)	Delaney	Maire (MOY-ruh)
Aisling (ASH-ling)	Eileen	Mairead (muh-RAID)
Aoife (EE-fuh)	Erin	Mamie
Brenna	Fallon	Maureen
Bridget	Fiadh (FEE-ah)	McKenna
Brigid (BRIH-jid)	Finley	Moira
Caoimhe (KEE-va)	Fiona	Molly
Casey	Flannery	Mona
Cassidy	Kathleen	Murphy
Ciara	Keira	Niamh (Neeve)
Clare	Kelly	Nora
Clodagh (CLOH-duh)	Kennedy	Oona
Colleen	Kerry	Orla

Quinlan	Ryan	Siobhan (shih-VONN)
Quinn	Saoirse (SEER-shuh)	Sloane
Reagan	Shannon	Sorcha (SOR-kuh)
Reilly	Shea	Tallula
Roisin (ro-SHEEN)	Sheridan	Teigan
Rory	Sinead (shih-NAID)	Tierney

BOYS

Aidan	Declan	Keir (Keer)	Rafferty
Aran	Dempsey	Kellen	Reilly
Brady	Dermot	Kevin	Rian (Ryan or REE-in)
Breccan	Dillon	Kieran	
Brendan	Donall	Kiernan	Riordan
Brennan	Donovan	Liam	Roark
Brian	Eamon	Lorcan	Ronan
Brogan	Ferris	Macauley	Rory
Callahan	Finley	Madden	Rowan
Carey	Finn	Maguire	Ryan
Casey	Finnegan	Murphy	Seamus (SHAY-mus)
Cian (KEE-in)	Finnian	Neil	Sean
Cillian	Fintan	Niall (Nile)	Shaw
Colin	Fitz	Nolan	Shay
Conall	Flynn	Oisin (oh-SHEEN)	Sullivan
Conan	Gallagher	Oscar	Tadhg ("tiger" without the "er")
Connelly	Gannon	Owen	
Connor	Gavin	Padraig (PAH drig)	Teague
Cormac	Grady		Torin
Crosby	Hartigan/Hart	Patrick	
Cullen	Hugh	Quinn	
Curran	Keegan		

Italian

There are millions of Italian Americans living in the US, many of whom want an Italian name that feels a bit more modern than classics like Tony or Angela. For boys, shorter names ending in vowels—like Enzo, Luca, and Matteo—have become popular. For girls, long feminine names ending in *a* like Isabella, Gianna, and Emilia have become stylish favorites. To really get creative, explore an Italian map for name inspiration: Sorrento (Ren), Capri, or Rome are a few ideas!

GIRLS

Adelina	Caterina	Giada	Maddalena
Alessandra	Chiara	Gianna	Marcella
Alessia	Concetta	Giulia	Mariella
Allegra	Cosima	Giuliana	Paola
Amara	Delfina	Ilaria	Pietra
Angela	Domenica	Imelda	Rafaella
Angelina	Edetta	Isabella	Renata
Antonella	Eloisa	Lelia	Serafina
Aria	Emilia	Leonora	Siena
Arianna	Emiliana	Lia	Teodora
Bella	Felice	Loretta	Toma
Bianca	Fiora	Lucia	Valentina
Bria	Francesca	Luciana	Via
Carina	Gabriella	Lucrezia	Violetta
Carla	Gemma	Luisa	Vivia
Carmela	Gia	Lunetta	Viviana

Aldo	Elio	Marco
Alessio	Enrico	Mario
Amato	Enzo	Massimo
Angelo	Filippo	Matteo
Aurelio	Francesco	Nero
Bosco	Franco	Nico
Brando	Gavino	Nicollo
Camillo	Giacomo	Oliviero
Carmelo	Gianni	Orso
Carlo	Giorgio	Remigio
Carmine	Giovanni	Rocco
Cassio	Giulio	Romeo
Cesco	Jacopo	Salvo
Ciro	Lando	Santino
Clemente	Leonardo	Taddeo
Cosimo	Lorenzo	Tommaso
Dante	Lucca	Tullio
Davide	Luciano	Vanni (short form
Dino	Lucio	of Giovanni)
Dominic	Marcello	Vincent

Latinx

A common request I get is for a name that would work both in America and in the client's family's country of origin, especially if they have relatives that speak a different language than English—most commonly Spanish. This is both a way to honor their heritage and a practical move that makes it easy to travel or live in another country where the name would blend right in. For parents looking to represent their Latino heritage or choose a name that works in a bilingual household, there are options like Elena, Isabella, Sophia, Santiago, Mateo, and Leonardo that have become very popular in America and now rank in the top 100. For somewhat more unique options that haven't quite taken off here yet, look to the most popular names being used in Spanish-speaking countries.

GIRLS

Adelina (Addy)	Claudia	Ines
Adriana	Dafne	Isabella (Isa, Bella)
Alba	Deisy	Jada
Alma	Dulce	Laia
Amada	Eleanora	Leticia (Leti)
Ana	Elena	Liliana (Lili)
Araceli (Celi)	Elodia	Lola
Avelina (Ava)	Emilia (Emi)	Lourdes (Lo, Lou)
Beatriz (Bea)	Esmeralda (Esme)	Lucia
Blanca	Eva (Evie)	Luciana (Luci)
Camila (Mila)	Flora	Luisa (Lu)
Carina (Nina)	Gabriela	Lupe
Carmen	Hilaria	Luz
Catalina (Lina)	Imelda	Maria

Marisol (Mari, Sol)	Ramona	Susana (Susy)
Marta	Reina	Valencia (Val/Cia)
Maya	Rosa (Rosie)	Valentina
Milagros (Millie)	Santana	Valeria
Natalia (Talia)	Selena	Verena (Vera)
Noelia (Noe)	Silvia (Silvie)	Vida
Pia	Sofia (Sofie)	Viviana (Vivi)
Pilar	Soledad (Sol)	Yesenia

BOYS

Adrian	Felipe	Luis
Alberto (Albi)	Fernando (Fernie)	Manuel
Alejandro (Ale)	Francisco (Frankie)	Marcello
Alonzo	Gael	Marco
Alvaro (Alvie)	Gonzalo (Zalo)	Martin (Marti)
Angel	Guillermo	Mateo (Teo)
Antonio	Hugo	Matias
Benicio (Benny)	Ignacio (Iggy)	Miguel
Camilo (Cam, Milo)	Inigo (Iggy)	Nico
Carlos	Jago	Nilo
Claudio	Jaime	Pablo
Clemente	Javier (Javi)	Pedro
Cristian	Joaquin (Quin)	Rafael (Rafa)
Cruz	Jorge	Rodrigo
Daniel	Jose	Santiago (Santi)
Diego	Leandro	Sergio
Eduardo (Edu)	Leonardo (Leo)	Tadeo
Emilio	Leonel (Leo)	Tavio (Tavi)
Enrique	Lorenzo (Enzo)	Teo
Esteban	Luca	Thiago

Literary

Literary names run the gamut; they can be classic, vintage, romantic, or eccentric. The names of some of your favorite fictional characters and authors can be a great source of name inspiration. Some people find inspiration in a recent bestseller (think Augustus and Hazel from *The Fault in Our Stars*, or Lily and Atlas from *It Ends with Us*). If there is a certain style of name you find yourself drawn to, like old money names, look up a list of the characters in *The Great Gatsby*. If you love more exotic names, flip through the A Court of Thorns and Roses series. Enjoy this list of names from some of the classics for the booklover naming a baby. **See also:** Soft and Poetic Boy Names.

GIRLS

Alice: *Alice in Wonderland*	Jane: *Jane Eyre*
Anne: *Anne of Green Gables*	Jo: *Little Women*
Cecily: *The Importance of Being Earnest*	Juliet: *Romeo and Juliet*
Charlotte (Charlotte Brontë)	Louisa (Louisa May Alcott)
Cosette: *Les Misérables*	Maya (Maya Angelou)
Daisy: *The Great Gatsby*	Ophelia: *Hamlet*
Darcy: *Pride and Prejudice*	Phoebe: *Catcher in the Rye*
Dorothy: *The Wonderful Wizard of Oz*	Poe (Edgar Allan Poe)
Edith (Edith Wharton)	Scarlett: *Gone with the Wind*
Eloise: *Eloise series*	Scout: *To Kill a Mockingbird*
Gwendolen: *The Importance of Being Earnest*	Toni (Toni Morrison)
Harper (Harper Lee)	Viola: *Twelfth Night*
Isolde: *Tristan and Isolde*	Virginia (Virginia Woolf)
	Zora (Zora Neale Hurston)

Arthur: *To Kill a Mockingbird*

Atticus: *To Kill a Mockingbird*

Austen (Jane Austen)

Bennett: *Pride and Prejudice*

Charles (Charles Dickens)

Finch: *To Kill a Mockingbird*

Fitz (F. Scott Fitzgerald)

George (George Orwell)

Gilbert: *Anne of Green Gables*

Harry: Harry Potter series

Holden: *The Catcher in the Rye*

Huck: *Adventures of Huckleberry Finn*

Hugo (Victor Hugo)

Huxley (Aldous Huxley)

Jack (Jack London)

Jay: *The Great Gatsby*

Jules (Jules Verne)

Leo (Leo Tolstoy)

Marlow: *Heart of Darkness*

Philip/Pip: *Great Expectations*

Quentin: *The Sound and the Fury*

Radley: *To Kill a Mockingbird*

Romeo: *Romeo and Juliet*

Salinger (J. D. Salinger)

Sawyer: *The Adventures of Tom Sawyer*

Sebastian: *Twelfth Night*

Theodore (Dr. Seuss's real first name was Theodor)

Tristan: *Tristan and Isolde*

Wilder (Laura Ingalls Wilder)

Winston: *1984*

Masculine/Gender-Neutral Names with Feminine Nicknames

We've seen that it's increasingly popular to give girls gender-neutral or even traditionally male names. If this trend appeals to you but you want a name that's more flexible, you might want to consider a masculine or gender-neutral name that easily nicknames to something traditionally feminine, like the names listed here, which can be used for any gender. **See also:** Boy Names for Girls, Feminine Names with Gender-Neutral Nicknames, Gender-Neutral, My Best Friend's Dad.

Ambrose: Rosie
Anderson: Andi
Anniston: Annie
Beckett: Beckie
Briar: Bri
Brookes: Brookie
Callan: Callie
Cameron: Cami
Campbell: Cami/ Bell
Conner: Coco
Dorian: Dori
Elliott: Elle/Ellie/ Lottie
Emmett: Emmy
Evan: Evie
Hollis: Hollie
Isaiah: Izzy

Jackson: Jackie
Jeremiah: Mia
Jonah: Joni
Julian: Jules
Lane: Lainey
Leighton: Lettie
Lennox: Leni
Linden: Linney
Logan: Lo, Loey
Luca: Lulu
Lucien: Lucy
Madden: Maddie
Magnus: Maggie
Mason: Maisie
Miles: Milly, Miley
Miller: Millie

Owen: Winnie

Penn: Penny

Reuben: Ruby

Riordan: Rio, Rory

Rome: Romy

Rudy: Rue

Spencer: Penny

Winslow: Winnie

Millennial

With millennials now becoming parents themselves (it's true, we're grown-ups), some are longing for the comfort and nostalgia of a familiar name, one that they heard during their childhood rather than the "new" names of today's top 100. While some names feel time-stamped because they were so common during the 1980s and '90s (Jessica, Brittany, and Jennifer for the girls, Jared and Kyle for the boys), some names survived and still feel relevant today. For girls, names like Meredith, Paige, and Brooke were prevalent but not overly popular and thus evaded a time stamp. For boys, names like Cameron, Blake, and Dylan retained their style and fit in among the boy (and girl!) names of today. If some of your fondest days were spent listening to *Spice* on your Discman while getting style inspo from *Seventeen* magazine and doodling with your milky gel pens, this list may just strike a chord. **See also:** Boomer Names, Refreshed; Surf, Skate, and Ski.

GIRLS

Alexandra	Brooke	Heather	Krista	Nicole
Alexis	Caitlin	Jacqueline	Laura	Paige
Alicia	Carly	Jamie	Lauren	Rachel
Allison	Carrie	Jasmine	Lindsey	Rebecca
Alyssa	Chelsea	Jennifer	Mallory	Sabrina
Amanda	Christine	Jessica	Megan	Samantha
Amber	Courtney	Jill	Melanie	Shelby
Amy	Danielle	Jordan	Melissa	Stephanie
Andrea	Emily	Kasey	Meredith	Sydney
Ashley	Erin	Kayla	Michaela	Taylor
Brianna	Haley	Kelsey	Michelle	Vanessa
Brittany	Hannah	Kimberly	Morgan	Victoria
			Natalie	

BOYS

Alex	Derek	Joshua
Austin	Devin	Justin
Blake	Dylan	Kevin
Bradley	Eric	Kyle
Brandon	Evan	Mark
Brendan	Garrett	Nathan
Brett	Gregory	Nicholas
Brian	Hunter	Patrick
Cameron	Ian	Ryan
Casey	Jacob	Scott
Chase	Jamie	Sean
Christian	Jared	Taylor
Christopher	Jason	Timothy
Cody	Jeff	Travis
Colby	Jeremy	Trevor
Corey	Jesse	Tyler
Daniel	Jordan	Zachary

Modern Cowboy/Cowgirl

These names range from mildly rustic to dashingly rugged. For boys, these are typically names that are distinctly masculine and feel bold and edgy. A tame choice here would be Wyatt or Walker (these can also lean private-school prepster), while something like Bridger or Bronco would be going the distance. Our modern cowgirl is not of the Dallas cheerleading variety but is instead a woman you might catch effortlessly wrangling cattle out on her Albuquerque ranch, or perhaps on the side of the road helping Brooks, who is on vacation with his family from upstate New York, change a tire. **See also:** Cool Girl Names, Edgy Boy Names.

GIRLS

Arizona	Hadley	Remington
Bellamy	Hazel	Ryder
Belle	Jessie	Sadie
Blakely	Jolene	Savannah
Brooklyn	Josie	Sedona
Cassidy	Kitt	Sierra
Chesney	Lainey	Stella
Cheyenne	Landry	Tess
Daisy	Liberty	Tilly
Dakota	Montana	Truett
Della	Nellie	Twyla
Delta	Oakley	Willa
Dolly	Rae	Winona
Georgia	Reba	Wyatt

BOYS

Ace	Hank	Rhett
Auburn	Harlan	Rhodes
Axel	Hart	Shepherd
Beau	Holt	Steele
Boone	Jackson	Sterling
Briggs	Jameson	Stetson
Bronco	Jennings	Stratton
Cade	Kit	Tanner
Cal	Knox	Tate
Cash	Lane	Tennessee
Cole	Lawson	Tex
Colt	Mac	Townes
Colter	Maverick	Trace
Dallas	Mills	Wade
Dax	Montgomery	Walker
Dempsey	Nash	Waylon
Denver	Radnor	West
Duke	Ramsey	Wilder
Dyer	Ranger	Wiley
Gentry	Reeve	Wyatt

More to Love

Looking to stand out instead of fit in? Trying to compromise with a partner who gets most of their name inspiration from Minecraft? "More to love" names draw from myth, fantasy, and stories set in other time periods. Often rooted in Latin, they retain a classical feel. These names feel big and bold, though often lend themselves to sweet nicknames, like Desi for Desdemona or Cal for Caledon. Multiple syllables and uncommon phonetic structures characterize these opulent, maximalist, a-little-bit-quirky names, which are pinnacles of creative expression and individuality. Many of these will turn heads at the playground. **See also:** Greek Mythology, Roman Mythology, Romantic.

GIRLS

Anastasia	Demetria	Flavia	Morwenna
Andromeda	Desdemona	Guinevere	Octavia
Antigone	Dorothea	Gwendolyn	Odessa
Apollonia	Drusilla	Hyacinth	Orianthe
Arcadia	Eleanora	Isadora	Peregrine
Artemis	Elfreda	Leonora	Persephone
Augusta	Esmeralda	Leticia	Philomena
Aurelia	Eugenia	Liviana	Seraphina
Calliope	Euphemia	Lucretia	Theodosia
Catalina	Evangeline	Lumina	Valentine
Cleopatra	Evanthe	Minerva	Wilhelmina
Cordelia	Evelith	Mirabella	Zenobia

BOYS

Alistair	Apollo	Augustus	Bartholemew
Aloysius	Archimedes	Aurelius	Bastien
Amadeus	Aristotle	Barnabas	Benedict

Caius	Florian	Marcellus	Severus
Caledon	Gulliver	Maximilian	Sylvester
Casimir	Horatio	Mordecai	Thaddeus
Cassius	Ignatius	Octavius	Titus
Constantine	Julius	Perseus	Ulysses
Cornelius	Leonidas	Percival	Valerian
Dante	Leopold	Phineas	Vergil
Darius	Lucius	Remegius	Wolfgang
Demetrius	Lysander	Rhysand	Xavier
Evander	Magnus	Santiago	Zacharius

My Best Friend's Dad

If traditional male names feel too masculine or formal to use for a girl, another option is using a traditionally male nickname. This list combines a few emerging trends: boy names for girls, nicknames as given names, and vintage comebacks. It sort of feels like you're naming your daughter after your childhood best friend's dad—Scott, Bill, Frank—but these names feel both sweet and edgy, traditional but unexpected. **See also:** Boy Names for Girls, Feminine Names with Gender-Neutral Nicknames, Gender-Neutral, Masculine/Gender-Neutral Names with Feminine Nicknames.

Andi	Denny	Kirby	Nicky	Scottie
Bennie	Frankie	Louie	Perry	Stevie
Billie	Freddie	Markie	Richie	Teddy
Bobbi	Georgie	Marty	Ricki	Terry
Charlie	Joey	Mattie	Robbie	Tommie
Davie	Johnnie	Mickey	Ronnie	Toni

Nature-Inspired

Did you know that Ari is Hebrew for "lion"? Or that Iris was the Greek goddess of rainbows? If you like names with a connection to nature but don't necessarily want to be as blatant as naming your child directly after a plant or animal, there are a number of subtler options to choose from. These names relate to the great outdoors through their meanings in mythology or other languages. **See also:** Celestial, Garden Glam, Outdoorsy.

GIRLS

Acadia: place-name	Goldie: color name
Aster: "star"	Ianthe: "purple flower"
Aurora: "dawn"	Iris: "rainbow"
Calanthe: "beautiful flower"	Luna: "moon"
Celeste: "heavenly"	McKinley: mountain
Ciel: "sky"	North: direction
Daphne: "laurel tree"	Nova: "new star"
Eden: biblical garden	Petra: "rock"
Eira: "snow" in Welsh	Selene: "moon"
Ember: "spark"	Seren: "star"
Estelle: "star"	Sierra: mountain range
Evanthe: "good flower"	Stella: "star"
Gaia: earth goddess	Terra: "earth"

BOYS

Adler: "eagle"	Beckett: "bee cottage"
Alder: "alder tree"	Calder: "rocky waters"
Ari: "lion"	Callum: "dove"
Arthur: "bear"	Clive: "cliff"
Aslan: "lion"	Corbin: "crow"
Banks: "edge of the river"	Darby: "deer park"

Easton: "east town"

Elio: "sun"

Everett: "strong boar"

Florian: "flower"

Ford: "river crossing"

Gray: color name

Harlan: "rocky land"

Heath: "stretch of open land"

Jonah: "dove"

Kai: "sea"

Leo: "lion"

Lochlan: "land of the lakes"

Lonan: "blackbird"

Murphy: "sea warrior"

Oliver: "olive tree"

Orson: "bear cub"

Rhodes: "where the roses grow"

Roscoe: "deer wood"

Silas: "of the forest"

South: direction

Sylvan: "of the forest"

Wesley: "west meadow"

Nickname Names

For some parents, regal names like Anastasia or Benedict, or even simple yet formal names like John or Anne, feel too "big" for a tiny baby. That's why many parents are now forgoing formalities and choosing a nickname as a given name, like Charlie instead of Charles or Millie instead of Amelia. Nicknames have a friendly and familiar feel. They often end in an *ee* sound that gives them a youthful and approachable vibe. Nicknames also offer a way to customize or modernize a family name being passed down, like Frankie for Frances or Ellie for Elizabeth. If you gravitate toward cuter names but have reservations about using one as a given name, go on a research rampage to figure out what formal names would get you to your desired nickname! For example, you could get the nickname Evie from Evelyn, Eve, Eva, Genevieve, Evangeline, Evette, Evelith, Evelina, Everly, Everett, Guinevere, Yvette, or even Eleanor Violet (E.V.). **See also:** Short and Sweet.

GIRLS

Addy	Cece	Esti
Ally	Coco	Evie
Andi	Daisy	Florie
Annie	Dolly	Flossie
Ari	Dory	Francie
Arlie	Dottie	Geri
Bessie	Dovie	Gertie
Betsy	Edie	Goldie
Betty	Effie	Gracie
Birdie	Ellie	Hattie
Bonnie	Elsie	Heidi
Bridie	Emmy	Hettie
Cassy	Essie	Izzy

Janie	Marley	Rosie
Jenny	Marnie	Ruby
Joey	Millie	Ruthie
Jolie	Minnie	Sadie
Jordy	Molly	Sosie
Josie	Nellie	Suki
Lainey	Noe	Sunny
Leni	Ori	Susie
Libby	Ottie	Sylvie
Lottie	Peggy	Tabby
Lulu	Penny	Tali
Maggie	Peri	Tedi
Maisie	Polly	Tilly
Mamie	Poppy	Winnie
Marcie	Posie	Zelie
Mari	Romy	Zuzu

BOYS

Albie	Jamie	Remy
Alfie	Joey	Richie
Archie	Johnny	Robbie
Ari	Jordy	Rory
Artie	Lenny	Rudy
Benji	Louie	Sammy
Billy	Matty	Tag
Charlie	Mickey	Teddy
Coby	Monty	Toby
Eddie	Ollie	Tommy
Frankie	Ozzy	Wally
Freddy	Pacey	Ziggy

Old Hollywood

Do you long for a bygone era of glamour and sophistication? Hollywood's golden age was characterized by dapper figures like Cary Grant and Clark Gable, Marilyn Monroe and Audrey Hepburn. The names on this list would be suitable for a *Great Gatsby*–themed party, with women in flapper dresses and feather boas and men sporting tailored pinstriped suits with fedoras, cigars in hand. This list is lively, luxurious, and timeless. **See also:** Cottage-core, Cozy by the Fire, Quiet Luxury.

GIRLS

Audrey	Helena	Marlene
Bette	Holly	Marnie
Blanche	Ingrid	Mimi
Blythe	June	Prudence
Clara	Kit	Rita
Claudette	Lana	Rooney
Constance	Lillian	Rosalind
Dagney	Lois	Roxie
Daisy	Lola	Scarlett
Dorothy	Louise	Simone
Florence	Lucille	Sinclair
Greer	Mamie	Violet
Greta	Marguerite	Virginia
Gwendolyn	Marilyn	Vivian

BOYS

Arthur	Bing	Claude
Atticus	Cary	Conrad
August	Clark	Darcy

Dashiell	Hugh	Pierce
Dean	Jay	Rex
Ellis	Kirk	Roy
Emerson	Kit	Sidney
Errol	Laurence	Simon
Frank	Leon	Spencer
Gable	Loren	Stanley
Gene	Lowell	Ted
Gilbert	Mackey	Thayer
Glenn	Monty	Truman
Guy	Orson	Vincent
Harvey	Oscar	Whit

Outdoorsy

If the first thing you put on your baby registry was an Osprey hiking backpack for your tot, you're going to want to take a look at this list. Some parents feel strongly about a first name that holds meaning, and nature can be a great source of inspiration! These also make for great middle names if they're a little outside of your first-name comfort zone. Some lean hippie (Fox, Finch), while some lean hipster (Atlas, Caspian). On the boys' side, some are earthy and gentle (River, Oak), and others are tough and masculine (Stone, Hawk). For girls, some nature names feel cool and edgy (Skye, Sol) while others feel tranquil and serene (Laurel, Meadow). Regardless, all of the names on this list reflect a connection to Mother Earth, and many are used for both genders. **See also:** Celestial; Free Spirit; Garden Glam; Nature-Inspired; Surf, Skate, and Ski.

GIRLS

Arbor	Minnow
Autumn	Pearl
Briar	Rain
Coral	Sable
Dove	Skye
Evergreen	Sol
Harbor	Solstice
Horizon	Starry
Lark	Summer
Laurel	Sunny
Maple	Vista
Marina	Winter
Meadow	Wren

Aire	Grove
Ash	Hawk
Aspen	Jetty
Atlas	Oak
Bear	Ocean
Birch	Phoenix
Bridger	Reed
Brooks	Reef
Canyon	Ridge
Cape	Rio
Caspian	River
Cedar	Robin
Cliff	Rocky
Coast	Sage
Comet	Shore
Cove	Slate
Cypress	Sonny
Dune	Spruce
Elm	Stone
Everest	Tide
Finch	Timber
Forest	Wilder
Fox	Wolf

Popular Names in Australia

Americans love to borrow ideas from effortlessly cool Aussies, so it's fun to take a look at name data from Down Under. Trends we see going strong in Australia include nicknames as given names, gender-neutral names, and royal family names. While there is a lot of overlap with the US, some names in Australia's top 100 that are not yet in America's top 100 include Eden, Elsie, Daisy, Florence, Frankie, Georgia, Margot, Matilda, Poppy, and Imogen for girls, and Archie, Alfie, Bodhi, Felix, Harvey, Hugo, Leon, Sonny, and Lochlan for boys. Below are the top 20 names for girls and boys in Australia from the most recent data in 2023. **See also:** Popular Names in the UK.

GIRLS

1. Isla	8. Willow	15. Isabella
2. Charlotte	9. Matilda	16. Evie
3. Olivia	10. Ella	17. Sophie
4. Amelia	11. Harper	18. Zoe
5. Ava	12. Chloe	19. Mila
6. Mia	13. Lily	20. Sophia
7. Grace	14. Ivy	

BOYS

1. Oliver	8. Theodore	15. Luca
2. Noah	9. Lucas	16. James
3. Jack	10. Thomas	17. Oscar
4. Henry	11. Elijah	18. Liam
5. William	12. Hudson	19. Alexander
6. Leo	13. Archie	20. Harrison
7. Charlie	14. Levi	

Popular Names in the UK

If you're the type of American who enjoys a crumpet with a cup of tea and wishes you were shopping for prams and nappies instead of strollers and diapers, you'll probably want to know about name trends in the United Kingdom. Luckily, the British government releases naming data for England and Wales every year. Much like in Australia, we see plenty of nicknames as given names, gender-neutral names, and royal family names. Some of the names that rank much higher in the UK than in the US include George, Muhammed, Arthur, Oscar, Archie, Arthur, Freddie, and Alfie for boys, and Freya, Florence, Sienna, Elsie, and Poppy for girls. Here are their top 20 names for girls and boys from 2023. **See also:** Popular Names in Australia.

GIRLS

1. Olivia	8. Florence	15. Elsie
2. Amelia	9. Isabella	16. Rosie
3. Isla	10. Mia	17. Grace
4. Ava	11. Willow	18. Millie
5. Lily	12. Sienna	19. Emily
6. Ivy	13. Poppy	20. Sofia
7. Freya	14. Sophia	

BOYS

1. Noah	8. Theodore	15. Harry
2. Muhammed	9. Theo	16. Charlie
3. George	10. Freddie	17. Alfie
4. Oliver	11. Archie	18. Arlo
5. Leo	12. Luca	19. Thomas
6. Arthur	13. Henry	20. Teddy
7. Oscar	14. Jack	

Positive Meaning

One way to start your child off on the right foot is to choose a name with a positive meaning. Who wouldn't be proud to sport a name with a meaning like "beauty" or "honor"? These girl and boy names bestow a beautiful message into your child's name, and many work well as middle names. (Keep in mind many names can have more than one meaning!) **See also:** Virtue Names.

GIRLS

Abigail: "Father's joy"

Agnes: "pure, holy"

Alice: "kind, noble"

Alma: "nourishing, soul"

Amanda: "worthy of love"

Amara: "everlasting"

Annora: "honor"

Arabella: "answered prayer"

Ariana: "most holy"

Beatrice: "bringer of joy"

Calla: "beauty"

Cara: "beloved, friend"

Carys: "love"

Celeste: "heavenly"

Claire/Clara: "bright"

Clementine: "merciful, gentle"

Diana: "heavenly, divine"

Eden: "paradise"

Elena: "shining light"

Emery: "brave"

Esme: "loved"

Evangeline: "good news"

Eve: "life"

Farrah: "happiness"

Felicity: "happiness"

Florence: "flowering, in bloom"

Freya: goddess of beauty, love, and fertility

Genevieve: "family woman"

Hannah: "grace"

Haven: "safe place"

Hillary: "cheerful, happy"

Imani: "belief, faith"

Irene: "peace"

Iris: "rainbow"

Jayce: "healer"

Jocelyn: "happy, joyful"

Karina: "love"

Katherine: "pure"

Kehlani: "sea heavens"

Leilani: "heavenly flower"

Lennon: "dear one"

Leticia: "joy"

Lior/Liora: "my light"

Lucy/Lucia: "of the light"

Luz: "light"

Mabel: "lovable"

Maya: "dream"

Nadia: "hope"

Naomi: "pleasant one"

Nora: "honor/shining light"

Pamela: "honey"

Philomena: "friend of strength"

Phoebe: "bright and pure"

Quinn: "wise"

Rowa: "lovely vision"

Ruth: "friend"

Sage: "wise"

Serena: "serene, calm"

Shiloh: "his gift"

Soloma: "peace"

Solveig: "sun strength"

Talia: "heaven's dew"

Uma: "splendor, tranquility"

Vera: "truth, faith"

Vivian: "alive"

Winifred/Wynn: "friend of peace, blessed"

Zoe: "life"

Zuri: "beautiful"

BOYS

Alden: "old friend"

Asa: "doctor, healer"

Asher: "happy, blessed"

Auden: "old friend"

Bennett: "blessed"

Caleb: "whole heart"

Callum: "dove"

Clement: "merciful"

David: "beloved"

Declan: "full of goodness"

Dorian: "gift"

Ellis: "kind and benevolent"

Emmett: "universal, truth"

Ethan: "strong, firm"

Ezra: "helper"

Felix: "happy"

Hugo: "mind, intellect"

Isaac: "laughter"

Jason: "healer"

Jonah/Jonas: "dove"

Jude/Judah: "praised"

Julian: "youthful, young at heart"

Kareem: "generous, giving"

Khalil: "friend"

Koda: "friend"

Levi: "joined in harmony"

Lucas/Lucius: "bringer of light"

Luke: "light-giving"

Mateo/Matthew: "gift from God"

Milo: "merciful"

Nathaniel: "gift of God"

Noah: "rest, comfort"

Rhys: "enthusiasm, passion"

Saul: "prayed for"

Sebastian: "venerable"

Sipho: "gift"

Soloman: "peace"

Tate: "cheerful"

Theodore: "gift of God"

Thomas: "twin"

Winston: "joyful stone"

Zane: "God's gracious gift"

Zayn: "beautiful"

Zorion: "happy"

Quiet Luxury

Quiet luxury emerged as a style trend in 2023 in the fashion industry and beyond. These names give off an understated elegance; they have subtle beauty and timeless appeal. If you're looking for a fresh take on the classics, this list has you covered. If you're looking for a name that passes the "Supreme Court test" (it would sound dignified on a justice), this list has you covered. They're sophisticated without being attention-grabbing—names like Desmond or Stuart rather than Kingston or Thaddeus. They're formal and serious, though many have the option of a more casual nickname. Still trying to get a grasp on the vibe? Imagine all of the neutral pieces from Kate Middleton's wardrobe; you've got quiet luxury. **See also:** French, Old Hollywood, Romantic, Soft and Poetic Boy Names, Traditional (with Nicknames).

GIRLS

Adair	Charlotte	Faye	Lenore
Agnes	Clara	Flora	Lucia
Anneliese	Claudia	Francesca	Margot
Astrid	Cosette	Gemma	Olivia
Audrey	Daphne	Genevieve	Penelope
Ava	Elise	Grace	Pippa
Beatrice	Elizabeth	Ingrid	Romilly
Bianca	Ella	Isabelle	Rosalie
Blythe	Eloise	Jane	Sabrina
Camille	Emilia	Josephine	Sophie
Carmen	Emma	Juliet	Talia
Cecilia	Esme	Justine	Vera
Celine	Esther	Kit	Vivienne

Adrian	Lawrence
Alden	Leland
Alexander	Louis
Arthur	Lucian
Atticus	Lyle
August	Malcolm
Clark	Oliver
Clement	Oscar
Conrad	Otto
Desmond	Perry
Gabriel	Phillip
Hugo	Sebastien
Jasper	Stuart
Julian	Theodore
Lance	Warren

Roman Mythology

Just like Greek mythology names, Roman mythology names offer a special balance between the traditional and the unique. Similar to virtue names or saints' names, these are names that seem to instill your child with positive symbolism or strength from the minute they arrive. This list will appeal to the history or mythology buff, or anyone who happens to be the former co-consul of their high school Latin club (guilty). **See also:** Celestial, Greek Mythology, More to Love, Romantic.

GIRLS

Aurora	Lavinia	Pomona
Bellona	Lucina	Rhea
Ceres	Lucretia	Salacia
Cybele	Luna	Silvia
Diana	Maia	Venus
Flora	Minerva	Vesta
Juno	Nemia	Victoria

BOYS

Albus	Gaius	Pax
Amadeus	Janus	Pluto
Apollo	Julius	Remus
Brutus	Jupiter	Romulus
Caelus	Mars	Silvius
Evander	Orcus	Vulcan

Romantic

Romantic girl names are elegant, feminine, beautiful, and poetic. They are often softer in sound; names that contain an l or end in an a abound on this list. Quite contrary to short, cool, gender-neutral girl names like Drew or Charley, romantic names may be longer and frillier. These are names that feel sweet but bold, fit for the main character of a fairy tale. They complement the idyllic image parents have of their unborn daughter, evoking love and optimism. Feminine but fiery, fresh but familiar. **See also:** French, Greek Mythology, More to Love, Quiet Luxury, Roman Mythology.

Alaia	Coralie	Helena	Melina
Alessia	Cosima	Ianthe	Natalia
Amalia	Delphine	Isabella	Nicola
Amara	Dorothea	Isobel	Odette
Amelie	Eliana	Isolde	Ophelia
Annelise	Eloise	Juliana	Paloma
Arabella	Emilia	Juliet	Portia
Arlette	Emmeline	Leisel	Rosalie
Aurelia	Esme	Leonora	Rosalind
Aurora	Evelina	Lilia	Selene
Aveline	Evianna	Liliana	Serafina
Bella	Fiona	Lilibet	Seraphine
Calista	Florence	Lisbet	Talla
Catalina	Francesca	Livia	Theodora
Cecily	Georgette	Lorelai	Valentina
Celeste	Giselle	Loretta	Vera
Charlene	Guinevere	Marceline	Violet
Charlize	Gwendolyn	Marguerite	Vivienne

Saints' Names

Choosing a saint's name for your child is typically rooted in Catholic naming tradition. Saints are revered figures who embody positive qualities or spiritual significance—perfect role models for your child. These names feel timeless, and many transcend cultural and linguistic boundaries. If none of the names on this list feel quite right, there are always ways to get creative. You could use a nickname like Remy instead of Remigius, or Rory instead of Gregory (both of which work for either gender). You could use Siena for a girl in honor of St. Catherine of Siena, or Aquinas with the nickname Quin in honor of St. Thomas Aquinas. You could use the surnames of saints, like Vianney or Campion, or you could use the feminine version of a traditionally masculine name, like Clementine for St. Clement. From steadfast traditional names like Anne and Luke to more distinctive names like Perpetua or Augustine, there is a spectacular spectrum of style amongst saints' names. **See also:** Biblical, Biblical (Bible Chic).

GIRLS

Adelaide	Catherine	Gianna
Agatha	Cecilia	Grace
Agnes	Celestine	Helena
Anastasia	Clare	Hilary
Anne	Colette	Hilda
Azelie	Edith	Hildegard
Barbara	Eleanor	Iris
Beatrice	Elizabeth	Jane
Bernadette	Frances	Jean
Bridget	Gemma	Joan
Camilla	Genevieve	Josephine

Julia	Magdalene		Rose
Kateri	Margaret		Siena
Louise	Mary		Teresa
Lucia	Matilda		Therese
Lucy	Perpetua		Veronica
Lydia	Philomena		Vivian (Bibiana)
Madeleine	Phoebe		

BOYS

Adrian	Cyril	Jude	Pius
Aidan	Damien	Kevin	Raphael
Alban	Dominic	Kolbe	Remigius
Alexander	Edmund	Lawrence	Robert
Ambrose	Edward	Leo	Sebastian
Anthony	Felix	Linus	Silas
Augustine	Fintan	Louis	Simeon
Benedict	Francis	Lucius	Simon
Bernard	Gabriel	Luke	Stephen
Blaise	George	Mark	Sylvester
Brendan	Gerard	Martin	Theodore
Bruno	Gregory	Maurice	Thomas
Charles	Henry	Maximilian	Timothy
Christopher	Hugh	Michael	Titus
Ciaran	Isaac	Nicholas	Valentine
Claude	James	Patrick	Victor
Clement	John	Paul	Vincent
Constantine	John Paul	Peter	Xavier
Cornelius	Joseph	Philip	

Scandinavian

Do you love a clean minimal look and want a baby name to match your interior design aesthetic? Scandinavian names originating in Denmark, Norway, and Sweden feel very stylish and could soon become more mainstream in the US, just as Irish, French, and Italian names have. For girls, names like Freya, Astrid, and Halle are in the top 1,000, and for boys, Axel and Magnus. Many Scandinavian boy names have a macho swagger (Viggo, Thor), while girl names can feel modern and feminine (Malin, Kaia). Using a Scandinavian surname like Andersen as a first name can work well too. Consider this list to find a baby name that feels just as hygge as your home.

GIRLS

Agnes	Elin	Lena
Alice	Ellinor	Linnea
Alva	Elsa	Liv
Anette	Freja	Lotte
Anneli	Freya	Lova
Annika	Greta	Malin
Asa	Halle	Mathilde
Astrid	Helene	Mille
Birgitte	Ingrid	Pia
Britta	Jensen	Signe
Dagmar	Juni	Sigrid
Dagny	Kaia	Solveig
Dahlia	Kajsa	Tuva

BOYS

Anders	Henrik	Milian
Andersen	Isak	Olle
Axel	Ivar	Oskar
Bengt	Kaj	Rune
Bernt	Kjell	Severin
Bjorn	Konrad	Soren
Casper	Larsen	Stellan
Einar	Leif	Sten
Erik	Lukas	Thor
Fredrik	Magnus	Torsten
Hans	Mikkel	Viggo

Short and Sweet

If you don't want to go too formal but also don't want to go too cute, short and sweet names occupy a great middle ground. They transcend age and feel fitting for both a child and an adult. These are (mostly) one- to two-syllable names that feel complete all on their own—no nickname needed. **See also:** Cool Girl Names, Nickname Names.

GIRLS

Abby	Eden	Ida	Lola
Ada	Edith	Ina	Lucy
Adele	Elise	Ines	Lula
Alba	Eliza	Iris	Luna
Alia	Ella	Isla	Lydia
Alice	Elle	Iva	Lyra
Alma	Elsa	Ivy	Mabel
Anna	Emma	Jane	Mae
Aria	Esme	Julia	Mara
Ava	Esther	Julie	Margot
Ayla	Etta	June	Marie
Bea	Eva	Kaia	Martha
Bella	Eve	Kate	Mary
Calla	Faye	Laure	Maya
Celia	Fern	Layla	Mia
Chloe	Flora	Leia	Mila
Claire	Gemma	Lena	Mira
Clara	Golda	Lia	Myla
Cora	Grace	Lila	Naya
Dahlia	Greta	Lily	Nell
Delia	Gwen	Lina	Nella
Della	Hallie	Liza	Noa

Noelle	Orla	Rosa	Uma
Nola	Pearl	Sela	Una
Nora	Petra	Sofia	Vera
Nyla	Pia	Stella	Willa
Olive	Pippa	Sybil	Xyla
Opal	Rhea	Tess	Zara
Ora	Roma	Thea	Zoe

BOYS

Arlo	Hayes	Noah
Axel	Heath	Penn
Bo	Hugh	Reese
Cal	Jack	Rhys
Clark	Jay	Rowan
Cole	Jude	Sage
Cy	Jules	Shay
Dane	Kai	Sol
Dean	Kit	Sonny
Des	Lane	Taj
Ellis	Leo	Tate
Finn	Liam	Theo
Fitz	Luca	Wade
Grey	Luke	Wynn
Gus	Milo	Zane
Harvey	Ned	Zev

Soft and Poetic Boy Names

This is a common style request for boy names—and it's a category I love! Think of this as the opposite of the macho cowboy names. These guys are gentle and sensitive. You could find them in the corner of their favorite speakeasy drinking a fernet and Coke, sporting a Carhartt beanie while purchasing a copy of *Walden* at their local used bookstore, or passionately protesting plastic straws outside Starbucks. Names like Ezra and Leo have already made it big, while Atlas and August are some of our rising stars. These names can lean indie, creative, or academic-sounding. **See also:** Literary, Quiet Luxury, Surnames as First Names (Old Soul).

Alaric	Everett	Oliver
Alistair	Ezra	Oren
Ansel	Franco	Otis
Arlo	Gideon	Pascal
Asa	Ira	Percy
Atlas	Isaiah	Perry
Atticus	Jasper	Robin
August	Julian	Rowan
Callum	Kit	Shay
Cy	Langston	Shiloh
Dashiell	Leo	Silas
Desmond	Lionel	Simon
Elias	Luca	Sol
Elijah	Lucien	Stel
Elliot	Marcel	Stellan
Ellis	Miles	Tobias
Emile	Milo	Tristan
Errol	Noah	Wilder

Surf, Skate, and Ski

Do you prefer to spend most of your time shredding waves or ski slopes? That may change temporarily with your new sidekick, but perhaps you want a name that fits your family's adventurous lifestyle! Think casual, cool and carefree kids wearing board shorts, Reef sandals, and a shark-tooth hemp necklace. If you're picturing the movie *Blue Crush*, we're on the same wavelength. My '90s kid bias is showing; this list definitely has a little bit of a '90s heartthrob vibe. **See also:** Millennial, Outdoorsy.

GIRLS

Alana	Cali	Harley	Leighton	Rae
Alex	Carly	Indi	Lexie	Riley
Aria	Cassidy	Jade	Lia	Sage
Aubrie	Coco	Jovie	Maren	Sam
Avery	Colbie	Juno	Marley	Siena
Blaire	Cory	Kaya	Morgan	Skye
Blake	Desi	Keely	Nicki	Summer
Bree	Hadley	Kylie	Paige	Sydney
Brooke	Hallie	Lainey	Perry	Teagan

BOYS

Adrian	Chase	Finn	Morgan	Sonny
Blake	Cody	Jake	Pacey	Tallon
Bodie	Crue	Jesse	Quinn	Tanner
Bowie	Dane	Kelly	Reese	Teague
Brig	Devin	Kieran	Riley	Tyler
Brody	Dillon	Layton	Rocky	Wes
Cal	Drew	Marley	Shane	Zack
Casey	Enzo	Miller	Slater	Zeke

Surnames as First Names

Using a surname as a given name is probably the most steadfast trend for both genders. Surnames are polished and established, yet fresh. Because they're names that have been around for so long, just not in the first-name slot, they often achieve that coveted label of "familiar but uncommon." There is an endless repository of surnames, so it's a great way to get creative with naming. It's nothing new; there are countless surnames in the top 100. What I expect to see is newer surnames entering the conversation, outside of the Carters, Coopers, Madisons, and Kennedys. Rhodes and Banks are on the rise for boys; Collins, Palmer, and Sutton are on the rise for girls. Names that are currently ranked very low that I have my eye on include Miller, Campbell, Jensen, Ellison, Lane, Murphy, Callahan, and Monroe. **See also:** Edgy Boy Names, Gender-Neutral, Surnames as First Names (Ivy League), Surnames as First Names (Old Soul).

Anderson	Bishop	Coleman	Dempsey
Anniston	Bradley	Collier	Doyle
Ashton	Brennan	Collins	Duncan
Austin	Bronson	Conlan	Easton
Bailey	Brooks	Conley	Elliot
Baker	Burke	Cooper	Ellis
Banks	Calder	Copeland	Evans
Barlow	Camden	Crosby	Fielder
Beale	Campbell	Daley	Fletcher
Beckett	Carson	Darby	Flynn
Beckham	Carter	Davis	Ford
Bennett	Channing	Dawson	Gannon
Benson	Cline	Dayton	Garrison
Berkley	Clinton	Decker	Garvey

Grady	Keller	Parker	Shaw
Grant	Kennedy	Pearson	Shepherd
Griffith	Kessler	Penn	Sinclair
Halston	Klein	Phalen	Smith
Harrison	Lavigne	Porter	Spencer
Hartley	Lennon	Presley	Stanton
Hayden	Lennox	Preston	Stiles
Hayes	Lincoln	Pruett	Stockton
Henderson	Mackey	Quinlan	Sullivan
Hendrix	Madison	Radley	Sutton
Henley	Mays	Ramsey	Taylor
Hewitt	Merrill	Redding	Tillman
Hudson	Merritt	Reed	Townes
Hunter	Miller	Reynolds	Truett
Jackson	Monroe	Rhodes	Tyson
Jacoby	Murphy	Riley	Wells
Jagger	Myers	Ripley	Weston
Jennings	Olson	Sanders	Winslow
Jensen	Palmer	Sawyer	York

Surnames as First Names (Ivy League)

Are you hoping to manifest a lifestyle of tennis at the country club, a summer home in the Catskills, and an Ivy League education? These luxurious-sounding surnames feel unique, classy, and wealthy. Whitaker might be seen interviewing for summer internships at the "Big Four," but if you see him out at a party you can just call him Whit. Nicknames like the ones I've listed alongside some of them (some more masculine, some more feminine) can give these proper names a more casual, friendly feel. As with all surnames, these work well as a given name for any gender. **See also:** Surnames as First Names, Surnames as First Names (Old Soul).

Aldrich

Beaumont (Beau)

Bentley (Ben)

Calloway (Cal, Clay)

Carlisle (Carli, Lyle)

Cavanaugh

Chamberlain (Lainey)

Chapman

Collins (Coco)

Copeland

Crawford (Ford)

Draper

Ellington (Ellie)

Elwood (Woody)

Emerson (Emmy, Sonny)

Fairfax

Fordham (Fordy)

Fraser (Fray)

Gallagher (Gal)

Hamilton (Millie)

Hardison (Hardy)

Hartwell (Hart, Wells)

Hastings

Hathaway

Hawthorne (Hawk)

Henning

Hillyard (Hilly)

Ingram (Gram)

Kennedy (Kenny)

Kensington (Kensie)

Kingsley

Lennox (Leni, Knox)

Lowell (Lo, Wells)

McCall (Mac, Mickey)

McKinley (Mac, Mickey, Kinley)

Merrick (Mere)

Monroe (Roe)
Osborne (Ozzy)
Pembroke (Pem)
Pennington (Penn, Penny)
Prescott (Scottie)
Preston
Quincy (Quin)
Rafferty (Rafe)
Richmond (Richie)
Schuyler (Sky)
Sinclair
Sumner

Tennyson (Tenn, Tenny)
Thompson (Thom)
Townsend (Townes)
Tripp
Truett (Tru)
Warner
Webster
Wellesley (Welles)
Westfield (West)
Whitaker (Whit)
Windsor (Winn, Winnie)
Yardley

Surnames as First Names (Old Soul)

This is another variation on the trend of using surnames as given names. "Old soul" surnames are not unlike "Ivy League" surnames, but they feel less preppy and more . . . liberal arts professor. This style often appeals to parents looking for something unique, vintage, soft, and gentle. **See also:** Surnames as First Names, Surnames as First Names (Ivy League), Soft and Poetic Boy Names.

Abbott	Ellis	Franklin	Marshall	Spencer
Clarke	Emery	Gibson	Murray	Stuart
Clary	Everett	Gordon	Nelson	Truman
Crosby	Ferguson	Graham	Reid	Vernon
Digby	Finnegan	Harris	Samson	Wallace
Edison	Foster	Irving	Sawyer	

Traditional (with Nicknames)

Traditional names are practical (less likely to be misspelled or mispronounced due to their universality) and often feel timeless as opposed to trendy. For parents looking for a name that will age well and avoid feeling dated, traditional names are often the place to look. I can't fight my love for a classic name with a cute, playful nickname. Especially on the boys' side, I get countless consults for classic-sounding names that are less common than Henry and Theodore or that haven't already been used by close friends or family. One of the best ways to have a fresh take on the classics is through creativity with nicknames, so I've included many in this list. **See also:** Biblical, Quiet Luxury, Vintage Darlings.

GIRLS

Abigail: Abby, Gail

Adeline: Addy, Della

Alice: Allie, Cece

Amelia: Emmy, Mia, Millie

Anna: Annie

Annabelle: Anna, Annie, Belle

Anne: Annie

Audrey

Bernadette: Berdie, Bernie, Etta, Bea

Bridget: Bridie

Caroline: Callie, Carrie, Linney, Roe

Cecilia: Cece, Ceci (Sessy), Celia

Charlotte: Charlie, Lottie

Claire

Eleanor: Elle, Ellie, Leni, Nellie, Nori, Nora

Elise: Ellie, Lise

Elizabeth: Elle, Ellie, Ella, Liza, Eliza, Libby, Beth, Betsy, Betty, Izzy, Birdie, Lizzy, Liz, Bea

Emily: Emmy, Millie

Esther: Essie, Esti

Eva: Evie

Frances: Fran, Francie, Frankie

Genevieve: Eve, Evie, Neve, Vivi, Gevie, Gen, Ginny

Grace: Gracie

Hannah

Harriet: Hattie

Isabelle: Izzy, Isa, Belle, Bella

Jane: Janie

Josephine: Josie, Joey, Jo, Effie

Julia: Julie, Jules

Katherine: Kate, Katie, Kit, Kat, Ren

Lillian: Lily/Lillie

Louisa: Lou, Lulu, Lo, Loey, Izzy

Lucy: Lulu

Madeline: Maddie, Mae, Della, Linney

Margaret: Daisy, Maggie, Maisie, Margo, Greta, Meg, Peg

Maria: Marie, Mari

Mary: Mae, Mamie

Rose: Rosie

Sophia: Sophie, Phia

Susanna: Susie, Sosie, Zuzu, Anna

Theresa: Tess, Tessa, Reese, Terry

Virginia: Vivi, Ginny, Gigi

BOYS

Adam

Alexander: Alex, Xander

Andrew: Andy, Drew

Arthur: Art, Artie, Bear (meaning of the name)

Benjamin: Ben, Benny, Benji

Charles: Charlie, Cal, Chuck

Christopher: Chris, Topher, Kit

Daniel: Dan, Danny

David: Dave, Davey

Edward: Eddie, Teddy, Ward

Frederick: Fred, Freddie, Fritz, Ricky

George: Geo, Georgie, Geordie

Henry: Hank

Isaac: Ike, Izzy, Zac, Ziggy

James: Jamie, Jay, Jimmy

John: Jack, Johnny, Jay

Joseph: Joe, Joey, JoJo

Lawrence: Law, Ren, Rence, Rory

Leo

Lewis: Lou

Luke

Matthew: Matt, Matty

Maxwell: Max, Wells

Michael: Mick, Mac, Mikey

Noah

Oliver: Ollie

Owen

Patrick: Pat, Paddy

Peter: Pete, Petey

Phillip: Phil, Flip, Pip

Robert: Rob, Robbie, Bobby, Bo, Bob, Bertie

Samuel: Sam, Sammy

Theodore: Teddy, Theo

Thomas: Tom, Tommy

Walter: Walt, Wally

William: Will, Billy, Liam

Unique

So you want to give your child a name that's unique—really unique. A guarantee they'll be the only one on their class list. Something that ranks outside not just the top 100 names but the top 1,000 names. None of the names listed here crack the top 1,000 (as of 2022, per SSA data); some are known, some are unusual, but they're all uncommon. **See also:** Influencer Names, Unique (1900).

GIRLS

Abilene	Bowie	Ellison
Adair	Brighton	Elowen
Adalie	Caitlin	Emmaline
Afton	Calla	Etta
Agnes	Cambria	Evelina
Alessi	Campbell	Ever
Amal	Cecily	Farrah
Ania	Chiara	Fern
Anouk	Coco	Francine
Arden	Colbie	Gaia
Auden	Colleen	Gala
Audra	Cordelia	Geneva
Aura	Corinne	Greer
Avalon	Courtney	Gwyneth
Azul	Danica	Halston
Baker	Darby	Harriet
Beatrix	Darcy	Hollis
Beckett	Delia	Ida
Bernadette	Eleni	Imogen
Betty	Ellery	Ines

Ingrid	Maeva	Seraphina
Irie	Maple	Seren
Isolde	Marjorie	Shai
Iva	Marnie	Shea
Jillian	Merritt	Sia
Joni	Micah	Solveig
Jude	Mildred	Sonia
Juno	Naia	Spencer
Kathleen	Nell	Sterling
Kiera	Nila	Story
Laia	Odette	Suri
Landry	Pepper	Sybil
Lane	Philippa	Tallulah
Lavender	Pia	Terra
Lavinia	Pippa	True
Leonie	Poet	Viola
Leonora	Polly	Wesley
Leora/Liora	Primrose	Whitney
Libby	Quincy	Winifred
Lilia	Reya	Winslow
Linden	Romy	Xena
Linnea	Rooney	Zaya
Lois	Rue	Zella
Lowen	Sable	Zia
Luca	Sally	Zinnia
Lula	Sedona	Zola
Lumi	Senna	Zyla

Alaric	Cormac	Gene	Lowen	Rush
Alastair	Cornelius	Geo	Lucien	Seamus
Angus	Cosmo	Glenn	Lyle	Shai
Anson	Cove	Guy	Mars	Shay
Aslan	Crawford	Hardy	Merrick	Simeon
Aspen	Crosby	Harlan	Niall	Smith
Auden	Cutler	Harris	Noam	Steele
Avett	Cypress	Hart	Noble	Stellan
Azai	Dashiell	Haze	Novian	Stockton
Basil	Dayton	Hollis	Oren	Stratton
Beck	Decker	Howard	Oslo	Tag
Bilal	Dempsey	Ignatius	Pacey	Taj
Bishop	Eamon	Iver	Paris	Townes
Blaise	Edmund	Jacoby	Pax	Trent
Boaz	Ellison	Jarvis	Penn	Truman
Brewer	Elvis	Jennings	Percy	Turner
Bronx	Ephraim	Judd	Perry	Vaughn
Caius	Ernest	Jules	Quade	Ward
Calder	Evren	Keller	Rafe	West
Campbell	Ferris	Kenai	Raleigh	Whitaker
Canyon	Finnian	Kent	Ranger	Wiley
Cedar	Finnick	Kip	Ransom	Willem
Cian	Fitz	Kit	Reef	Woodrow
Clement	Foster	Leander	Rennick	Zealand
Cline	Fox	Lev	Ripley	Zephyr
Clive	Frey	Lex	Rook	Zeus
Coleman	Gannon	Link	Roscoe	Zev
Colsen	Garrison	Locke	Rune	Ziggy

Unique (1900)

With many vintage names having a comeback, some are starting to lose the fresh and unexpected appeal that parents are looking for as they become mainstream on playgrounds and in preschools. If you're looking for a particular kind of vintage name, one with a certain unique flair, look no further. The names listed here were in the top 1,000 in the year 1900 but have fallen in popularity since then, making them perfectly ripe for a refresh. **See also:** Unique, Vintage Darlings, Vintage Grandma and Grandpa.

GIRLS

Alva	Eulalia	Golda	Luvenia	Rhoda
Alvera	Eunice	Ina	Melba	Roxie
Beulah	Flossie	Ines/Inez	Minerva	Sybil
Elnora	Freda	Iola	Nanette	Velma
Elva	Geneva	Iva	Nettie	Wilhelmina
Eula	Geraldine	Lela	Ora	Zula

BOYS

Abner	Dudley	Homer	Monroe
Anton	Elmer	Horace	Monty
Aubrey	Elton	Ike	Myron
Booker	Elwood	Leroy	Percy
Boyd	Erwin	Leslie	Roland
Carroll	Freeman	Lester	Roscoe
Cecil	Grover	Lonnie	Sterling
Clair	Hardy	Loren	Vernon
Cornelius	Harley	Maynard	Wendell
Delbert	Herman	Merle	Willard
Dewey	Herschel	Milton	Wilmer

Vintage Darlings

Do you plan on dressing your child in Peter Pan collars and Mary Janes, adorning their nursery with antique frames and Grandma's old quilt? Then vintage names may be for you. Some are more charming (these feel more modern, already having made a comeback), while others are more on the elegant side (these feel like they belong to your mother-in-law who uses the family china for a Monday night dinner), but all bring a timeless appeal to the table. **See also:** Cottagecore, Traditional (with Nicknames), Unique (1900), Vintage Grandma and Grandpa.

GIRLS

Adelaide	Florence	Mae
Alice	Frances	Maisie
Beatrice	Goldie	Mamie
Blanche	Gussie	Marion
Celia	Hattie	Martha
Clara	Hazel	Mattie
Constance	Iris	Maude
Cora	June	Millie
Daisy	Lettie	Minnie
Delia	Lillian	Nellie
Della	Lois	Olive
Delphine	Lola	Pearlie
Dottie	Lottie	Rose
Eleanor	Louisa	Ruby
Elsie	Louise	Sallie
Etta	Lucille	Scarlett
Evelyn	Luella	Sylvie
Faye	Lula	Tessie
Flora	Mabel	Thea

Tillie	Viola	Virginia
Vera	Violet	Vivian

BOYS

Albert	Ferris	Leon
Alfred	Francis	Linus
Arlo	Franklin	Louis
Arthur	Frederick	Ollie
Artie	George	Orson
Calvin	Gus	Oscar
Carey	Guy	Otis
Charles	Hal	Otto
Dale	Hank	Rexford
Dean	Harvey	Sidney
Edmund	Hugh	Simon
Ellis	Hugo	Walter
Emory	Jasper	Ward
Everett	Laurence	Wesley
Felix	Leo	Winston

Vintage Grandma and Grandpa

Now that we're getting used to seeing vintage names, some parents want to go even further, digging through the archives to rediscover outdated vintage names. This is a great way to stick to an on-trend category but branch out to more unique names within that category. If these names had a smell, it would be that of an antique bookstore; if they had a sound, it would be the crackling of a vinyl record. A little bit comfortable, a little bit bold, they evoke a bygone era with old-school style. **See also:** Cottagecore, Unique (1900), Vintage Darlings.

GIRLS

Agatha	Hilda
Agnes	Ida
Alma	Jemima
Althea	Joan
Anita	Marjorie
Arlene	Mildred
Betty	Millicent
Bonnie	Myra
Cornelia	Nell
Doris	Opal
Dorothea	Pauline
Dorothy	Pearl
Edith	Rita
Edna	Ruth
Estelle	Sally
Ethel	Shirley
Gladys	Sylvia
Helen	Thelma
Henrietta	Winifred

Allen	Luther
Alvin	Lyle
Arnold	Martin
Baxter	Maurice
Bernard	Melvin
Bruce	Ned
Claude	Norman
Clifford	Ralph
Earl	Ray
Elmer	Reuben
Ernest	Roger
Floyd	Roy
Gene	Russell
Gilbert	Seymour
Glenn	Stanley
Gordon	Sylvester
Harold	Wade
Herbert	Wallace
Howard	Warren
Leonard	Wilfred

Virtue Names

When we think of "virtue names," we usually think of historically mainstream names like Grace, Hope, or Faith. These days, more unique virtue names are on the list of fastest-rising baby names, including Chosen and True for boys and Blessing and Promise for girls. These names appeal to parents who want their child's name to align with cultural or spiritual values they hold or simply to elicit a positive association or meaning. Here is a short list of wearable, fresh virtue names to consider for your baby! **See also:** Positive Meaning.

GIRLS

Essence	Poet
Felicity	Reverie
Haven	Sage
Honor	Solace
Love	True
Merritt	Verity

BOYS

Brave	Noble
Clement	Pax
Creed	Valor
Earnest	Wit
Hero	Worth
Merit	Zen

10 Most Popular Names
by Decade

We'll close with a list of the top 10 names at the start of each decade according to SSA data, beginning in the year 1900. This can be a great way to find inspiration from the past or just to observe the way naming trends have come and gone over the past hundred-plus years. Whether you're excited to have your kids join the ranks of Liams and Olivias or you aspire to bring back Frank and Florence, these names are a fascinating time capsule!

1900

GIRLS

1. Mary	6. Elizabeth
2. Helen	7. Florence
3. Anna	8. Ethel
4. Margaret	9. Marie
5. Ruth	10. Lillian

BOYS

1. John	6. Robert
2. William	7. Joseph
3. James	8. Frank
4. George	9. Edward
5. Charles	10. Henry

1910

GIRLS

1. Mary	6. Anna
2. Helen	7. Elizabeth
3. Margaret	8. Mildred
4. Dorothy	9. Marie
5. Ruth	10. Alice

BOYS

1. John	6. Joseph
2. James	7. Charles
3. William	8. Frank
4. Robert	9. Edward
5. George	10. Henry

1920

GIRLS

1. Mary	6. Mildred
2. Dorothy	7. Virginia
3. Helen	8. Elizabeth
4. Margaret	9. Frances
5. Ruth	10. Anna

BOYS

1. John	6. George
2. William	7. Joseph
3. Robert	8. Edward
4. James	9. Frank
5. Charles	10. Richard

1930

GIRLS

1. Mary	6. Barbara
2. Betty	7. Patricia
3. Dorothy	8. Joan
4. Helen	9. Doris
5. Margaret	10. Ruth

BOYS

1. Robert	6. Charles
2. James	7. Donald
3. John	8. George
4. William	9. Joseph
5. Richard	10. Edward

1940

GIRLS

1. Mary	6. Carol
2. Barbara	7. Nancy
3. Patricia	8. Linda
4. Judith	9. Shirley
5. Betty	10. Sandra

BOYS

1. James	6. Charles
2. Robert	7. David
3. John	8. Thomas
4. William	9. Donald
5. Richard	10. Ronald

1950

GIRLS

1. Linda
2. Mary
3. Patricia
4. Barbara
5. Susan
6. Nancy
7. Deborah
8. Sandra
9. Carol
10. Kathleen

BOYS

1. James
2. Robert
3. John
4. Michael
5. David
6. William
7. Richard
8. Thomas
9. Charles
10. Gary

1960

GIRLS

1. Mary
2. Susan
3. Linda
4. Karen
5. Donna
6. Lisa
7. Patricia
8. Debra
9. Cynthia
10. Deborah

BOYS

1. David
2. Michael
3. James
4. John
5. Robert
6. Mark
7. William
8. Richard
9. Thomas
10. Steven

1970

GIRLS

1. Jennifer	6. Angela
2. Lisa	7. Melissa
3. Kimberly	8. Tammy
4. Michelle	9. Mary
5. Amy	10. Tracy

BOYS

1. Michael	6. Christopher
2. James	7. William
3. David	8. Brian
4. John	9. Mark
5. Robert	10. Richard

1980

GIRLS

1. Jennifer	6. Heather
2. Amanda	7. Nicole
3. Jessica	8. Amy
4. Melissa	9. Elizabeth
5. Sarah	10. Michelle

BOYS

1. Michael	6. Matthew
2. Christopher	7. Joshua
3. Jason	8. John
4. David	9. Robert
5. James	10. Joseph

1990

GIRLS

1. Jessica	6. Sarah
2. Ashley	7. Stephanie
3. Brittany	8. Jennifer
4. Amanda	9. Elizabeth
5. Samantha	10. Lauren

BOYS

1. Michael	6. David
2. Christopher	7. Andrew
3. Matthew	8. James
4. Joshua	9. Justin
5. Daniel	10. Joseph

2000

GIRLS

1. Emily	6. Alexis
2. Hannah	7. Samantha
3. Madison	8. Jessica
4. Ashley	9. Elizabeth
5. Sarah	10. Taylor

BOYS

1. Jacob	6. Nicholas
2. Michael	7. Andrew
3. Matthew	8. Joseph
4. Joshua	9. Daniel
5. Christopher	10. Tyler

2010

GIRLS

1. Isabella	6. Emily
2. Sophia	7. Abigail
3. Emma	8. Madison
4. Olivia	9. Chloe
5. Ava	10. Mia

BOYS

1. Jacob	6. Alexander
2. Ethan	7. Noah
3. Michael	8. Daniel
4. Jayden	9. Aiden
5. William	10. Anthony

2020

GIRLS

1. Olivia	6. Amelia
2. Emma	7. Isabella
3. Ava	8. Mia
4. Charlotte	9. Evelyn
5. Sophia	10. Harper

BOYS

1. Liam	6. James
2. Owen	7. Benjamin
3. Oliver	8. Lucas
4. Elijah	9. Henry
5. William	10. Alexander

acknowledgments

First and foremost, I'd like to thank my husband, Dan, who has been my biggest encourager and supporter through this naming venture. Truly would not be here without you.

I want to thank my friends and family for sharing the joy in this dream come true. My parents, siblings, and cousin squad who fueled this fire at a young age. And my friends for the endless, endless name chats.

I want to thank the team at Tarcher, especially my editor, Lauren O'Neal, who was paramount in bringing this vision to fruition and always made me feel like adding "author" to my résumé wasn't that crazy.

Finally, I want to thank all my fellow name nerds and readers who will pick up this book. I never knew there were so many of us out there who share such a passion for names. I am so thankful for your support and engagement; this would not have been possible without you!

notes

Chapter 1

8 **Puritans in seventeenth-century:** Joseph Norwood, "A Boy Named Humiliation: Some Wacky, Cruel, and Bizarre Puritan Names," *Slate*, September 13, 2013, https://slate.com/human-interest/2013/09/puritan-names-lists-of-bizarre-religious-nomenclature-used-by-puritans.html.

Chapter 2

22 **The names Allison, Leslie:** "It's a Boy! Now, It's a Girl! 8 Baby Names That Switched Genders," Ancestry.com, September 8, 2014, https://www.ancestry.ca/c/ancestry-blog/its-a-boy-now-its-a-girl-8-baby-names-that-switched-genders.

23 **Did you know that Cameron:** Name meanings here and elsewhere are taken from behindthename.com.

Chapter 3

45 **In New Zealand in 2023:** Rachel Paula Abrahamson, "New Zealand Has a Long List of Banned Baby Names—and American Parents Wouldn't Be Happy," Today.com, January 26, 2024, https://www.today.com/parents/family/new-zealand-banned-baby-names-rcna135625.

48 **According to the website:** "Name Popularity," Our Baby Namer, accessed January 9, 2025, https://www.ourbabynamer.com/name-popularity.html.

53 **Even in the 1700s:** Clive Thompson, "The Science of Baby-Name Trends," JSTOR Daily, December 28, 2019, https://daily.jstor.org/science-baby-names.

Chapter 5

86 **As baby name expert:** Sophie Kihm, "Twin Names: The Ultimate Guide," Nameberry, August 24, 2024, https://nameberry.com/blog/twin-names-the-ultimate-guide.

93 **As Kihm writes:** Sophie Kihm, "How to Cope with Baby Name Regret," Nameberry, October 26, 2023, https://nameberry.com/blog/baby-name-regret.

102 **Beyond these entertaining associations:** Marianne Bertrand and Sendhil Mullainathan, "Are Emily and Greg More Employable than Lakisha and Jamal? A Field Experiment on Labor Market Discrimination," *American Economic Review* 94, no. 4 (2004): 991–1013, DOI: 10.1257/0002828042002561.

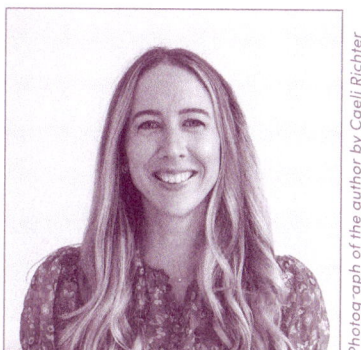

Colleen Slagen is a professional baby name consultant and content creator. A former nurse practitioner, she launched her business, Naming Bebe, in 2021. Since then, her social media content has reached an audience of millions of people worldwide, and her work has been featured on NPR, ABC News, *Today*, *The Washington Post*, and more. She lives in the Boston area with her three children and her husband, who never, ever grows tired of chatting about baby names.